REVERSE TYPE 2 DIABETES DIET

INCLUDES 30-DAY MEAL PLAN, BEST AND WORST FOODS, AND AN EXTENSIVE 4000+ FOOD LIST RANKED BY GI, GL, AND CARB GRAMS

DR. H. MAHER

CONTENTS

PREFACE

In our modern era, a silent pandemic is sweeping across the globe. Type 2 Diabetes (T2D), once considered an unavoidable fate, is rapidly escalating. In 2019, its prevalence was estimated at 9.3% (463 million people), and projections suggest an alarming rise to 10.9% (700 million) by 2045. Furthermore, the strong link between obesity and T2D is indisputable, with up to 90% of individuals diagnosed with T2D being overweight or obese. This growing crisis demands immediate attention and decisive action.

T2D is not a standalone condition—it wreaks systemic havoc, leading to devastating complications that can affect every part of the body. Its prevalence is, in part, a result of the widespread adoption of Western dietary patterns, which typically consist of high-fat, high-sugar, and refined foods, while being deficient in essential nutrients. The implications of this dietary trend extend beyond T2D, contributing to an array of degenerative and chronic diseases.

However, amid this gloom, a glimmer of hope emerges. Rigorous scientific research and our growing understanding of the disease now suggest that T2D can be potentially reversed. Thanks to ground-breaking work, such as Taylor's Twin Cycle Hypothesis, we've come to understand that T2D often results from excessive fat accumulation in the liver and pancreas.

Leading health organizations, including the American Diabetes Association (ADA), the Endocrine Society, and the European Association for the Study of Diabetes (EASD), now define T2D remission as a return to normal blood glucose levels for at least three months without any glucose-lowering pharmacotherapy. This substantial shift in understanding is revolutionary, signaling a profound change in our approach to managing and treating T2D.

Despite these advances, reliance on pharmacotherapy alone is insufficient and often associated with side effects. While medication plays a significant role, especially insulin and certain diabetes medications like sulfonylureas and thiazolidinediones, addressing the underlying unhealthy lifestyles and promoting weight loss are equally critical. Unfortunately, current guidelines for T2D management often fall short of emphasizing these crucial lifestyle factors.

That's where "Reverse Type 2 Diabetes Diet" steps in. This book marries extensive scientific knowledge, experiential wisdom, and effective nutritional strategies into a comprehensive, user-friendly guide. It offers a practical, evidence-based path forward, using the principles of the Mediterranean diet, the Glycemic Index-Glycemic Load (GI-GL) framework, and the 2020-2025 Dietary Guidelines for Americans.

By fostering empowerment, we aim to equip you with the knowledge and tools you need to make confident dietary choices and steer your health in the right direction. The journey towards health improvement and potential T2D reversal can be complex, but we aim to simplify it.

Join us on this transformative journey, as we provide practical 30-day meal plans, outline the seventeen principles of the Reverse Type 2 Diabetes Diet, and compile an extensive list of foods, complete with serving sizes, Glycemic Index, Glycemic Load, and net carbohydrates data. Let this book be your guiding light on the path to restored health and wellness.

Yours in health,

Dr. H. Maher

Dr. Y. Naitlho, PharmD

H. Naitlho, MEng (ISAE-SUPAERO), MEng (École de l'Air), MSc (Paul Sabatier University), EMBA

INTRODUCTION

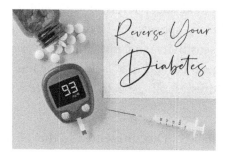

Are you looking for a comprehensive, multi-dimensional dietary approach that transcends traditional advice for managing or even reversing Type 2 Diabetes? Do you aspire to join the growing number of people who have triumphed over their T2D? This book offers you powerful tools, grounded in the latest dietary principles of the Mediterranean diet, the glycemic index, and glycemic load framework, alongside cutting-edge health and nutrition science. Together, these elements converge into Reverse Type 2 Diabetes Diet, promoting optimal weight management and fostering long-term improvements in insulin sensitivity - two key factors in effectively managing and potentially reversing Type 2 Diabetes. This comprehensive guide is your passport to a healthier journey toward achieving these life-changing goals.

Introduction to Type 2 Diabetes and Reversal Approaches

Type 2 diabetes (T2D) is a widespread and severe metabolic disorder that currently affects approximately 540 million adults aged 20 to 79 years globally. This chronic condition is marked by elevated blood sugar levels, insulin resistance, and a deficiency of insulin to varying degrees. If left uncontrolled, T2D can progress to serious health complications such as chronic kidney damage, heart disease, neuropathy, and vision loss. Moreover, it substantially increases the likelihood of experiencing a stroke and premature mortality.

One crucial aspect of managing T2D is diet, as the food we consume directly impacts blood sugar levels, body weight, and overall well-being. Certain dietary approaches have even shown the potential to enhance insulin sensitivity and potentially reverse T2D. However, until recently, there has been a lack of a comprehensive dietary strategy that addresses all aspects of diabetes management and reversal.

Reverse Type 2 Diabetes Diet, presented in this book, aims to bridge this gap. This innovative and scientifically-supported approach combines principles from successful diets and the latest nutritional research, providing a holistic solution to manage and potentially reverse T2D. By incorporating the best practices from various dietary approaches, this diet offers a comprehensive and individualized plan to support people with T2D in achieving better health outcomes, and ultimately reversing diabetes.

The Twin Cycle Hypothesis

The Twin Cycle Hypothesis, from Professor Roy Taylor and his team, explains how Type 2 diabetes starts. It points to a harmful cycle in the liver and pancreas. Initiated by excessive consumption of high-calorie, high-fat, and high-sugar foods, surplus fat accumulates in the liver, leading to hepatic steatosis. This results in elevated blood glucose levels and increased insulin production, eventually causing pancreatic fat buildup and beta cell dysfunction.

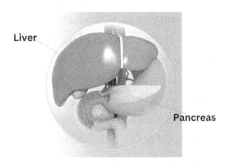

The importance of the Twin Cycle Hypothesis lies in its illumination of the path to reversing type 2 diabetes. It suggests that cutting down on high-calorie, high-fat, and high-sugar foods, and encouraging the consumption of nutrient-rich, low-glycemic, high-fiber alternatives could reverse the disease. That's precisely where Reverse Type 2 Diabetes Diet comes in. By curbing the intake of these harmful foods and fostering healthier eating patterns, it assists in eliminating excess fat from the liver and pancreas, boosts insulin sensitivity, and holds the potential to halt or even reverse the disease's progression.

What is Reverse Type 2 Diabetes Diet?

Reverse Type 2 Diabetes Diet is an innovative, integrated dietary approach designed to effectively manage and target type 2 diabetes. It combines successful principles from various dietary strategies, the latest nutritional research, and presents them in a cohesive, and easy-to-follow format.

Reverse Type 2 Diabetes Diet has three core components:

- **Glycemic Index (GI) and Glycemic Load (GL)**

Principles: The Glycemic Index and Glycemic Load are valuable tools used to assess the impact of foods on blood sugar levels. The GI assigns a score to foods, indicating how rapidly they raise blood sugar compared to a reference food like glucose or white bread. However, the GI alone does not account for the quantity of carbohydrates in a food portion, which is where the GL comes into play. The GL considers both the quality and quantity of carbohydrates, offering a more comprehensive understanding of how a food affects blood sugar levels.

- **Mediterranean Diet (MedDiet) Principles:** The MedDiet is one of the world's most researched and praised diets, known for its heart-healthy and weight-managing benefits. Reverse Type 2 Diabetes Diet borrows key components from this dietary pattern, such as emphasizing the consumption of whole grains, fruits, vegetables, lean proteins, healthy fats, and minimally processed foods.

- **2020-2025 Dietary Guidelines for Americans:** These guidelines provide advice on healthy eating patterns to promote health, prevent chronic diseases, and maintain a healthy weight. Reverse Type 2 Diabetes Diet is designed to align with these guidelines, encouraging the consumption of nutrient-dense foods rich in essential vitamins, minerals, and other beneficial compounds, while being relatively low in calories.

Pulling it all together, Reverse Type 2 Diabetes Diet incorporates these principles to create a comprehensive dietary approach. By consuming nutrient-dense, low-glycemic foods and controlling portions, you can balance your food intake, avoid blood sugar spikes, manage your weight, and potentially reverse type 2 diabetes. This diet not only encourages the reduction of highly processed foods, which often contain unhealthy fats, sugars, and sodium, but also promotes an increased intake of nutritionally dense alternatives.

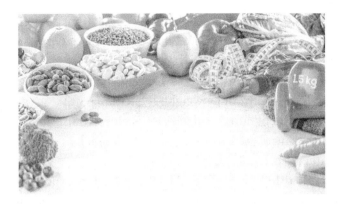

Empirical Evidence Supporting Reverse Type 2 Diabetes Diet

Reverse Type 2 Diabetes Diet's effectiveness is backed by empirical research and clinical trials. These studies affirm the positive effects of the Glycemic Index (GI), Glycemic Load (GL), and Mediterranean Diet principles on type 2 diabetes management. Details of these studies will be discussed extensively in the forthcoming chapters.

Benefits of the Reverse Type 2 Diabetes Diet

Reverse Type 2 Diabetes Diet provides potential benefits for individuals diagnosed with type 2 diabetes, as well as those who face a risk of developing the condition or those who simply want to enhance their overall health.

- **Improved Blood Sugar Control:** Following Reverse Type 2 Diabetes Diet leads to better control of blood glucose levels. The diet prioritizes foods with low Glycemic Index and Glycemic Load, which help prevent rapid blood sugar spikes and promotes overall glycemic control.
- **Potential Diabetes Reversal:** Early research suggests that following Reverse Type 2 Diabetes Diet, in combination with regular exercise and weight loss, could ultimately lead to the remission of type 2 diabetes. The diet is designed to help

'reset' your body's insulin and glucose regulation, potentially reversing the metabolic issues that contribute to type 2 diabetes.

- **Weight Management:** Reverse Type 2 Diabetes Diet promotes a healthy body weight. It encourages the consumption of nutrient-dense, low-calorie foods, and portion control, which can assist with weight loss or weight maintenance.
- **Heart Health:** Reverse Type 2 Diabetes Diet incorporates principles from the Mediterranean Diet, which is renowned for its heart-healthy benefits. These include lowering cholesterol levels and reducing the risk of heart disease.
- **Enhanced Nutritional Intake:** By prioritizing nutrient-rich foods, the diet substantially enhances your overall nutrient intake. It simultaneously encourages limiting consumption of heavily processed foods, typically laden with unhealthy fats, sugars, and sodium, thereby fostering a healthier nutritional balance.
- **Lowered Risk of Additional Chronic Diseases:** The principles underpinning Reverse Type 2 Diabetes Diet not only aid in managing type 2 diabetes, but they also correlate with a reduced risk of various other chronic diseases. This nutritional approach is associated with a decreased likelihood of conditions such as heart disease, certain types of cancer, and hypertension.
- **Flexibility and Sustainability:** Reverse Type 2 Diabetes Diet is not restrictive; rather, it promotes a balanced approach to eating. It allows for a wide variety of foods, making it easier to stick to in the long term compared to restrictive diets.

What to Expect from This Book

As you delve into this comprehensive guide, you can anticipate a well-rounded, scientifically-backed, and practical approach to managing and potentially reversing type 2 diabetes through diet. Here is a quick snapshot of what you can expect:

- **Comprehensive Understanding:** The book first educates you about type 2 diabetes, its causes, and the importance of dietary interventions. We've explained complex concepts in simple language, making them easy for anyone to understand, whether or not they have a medical background.
- **Science-Based Approach:** We delve into the science behind Reverse Type 2 Diabetes Diet, including the Twin Cycle Hypothesis, the principles of the Glycemic Index (GI) and Glycemic Load (GL), and the health benefits of the Mediterranean Diet. All recommendations are rooted in the latest scientific research.
- **Practical Tools:** The book provides practical tools such as meal plans, food lists, and expert meal planning. It offers a roadmap on how to implement Reverse Type 2 Diabetes Diet in your daily life.
- **Customization Tips:** We understand that everyone's nutritional needs and preferences are unique. Thus, we offer advice on how to personalize Reverse Type 2 Diabetes Diet to align with your lifestyle, food preferences, and specific health needs.
- **Evidence-Based Benefits:** You'll learn about the evidence supporting Reverse Type 2 Diabetes Diet, the research that validates its principles, and the potential benefits of adopting this diet.
- **Ongoing Support:** The book also includes strategies to help you stick to the diet long-term and integrate it into your lifestyle. We've added tips to overcome common challenges and maintain motivation.

* * *

Embrace the journey towards a healthier you, today. Don't wait to make the lifestyle changes necessary to reverse type 2 diabetes, avoid life-threatening complications, and achieve optimal weight. Start by turning the page and stepping into the world of the Reverse Type 2 Diabetes Diet. Remember, each step you take is not just towards managing diabetes, but potentially reversing it entirely. The power to change your life is in your hands. Start your transformative journey now!

PART I
FOUNDATIONS OF THE TYPE 2 DIABETES REVERSAL DIET: UNDERSTANDING THE SCIENCE

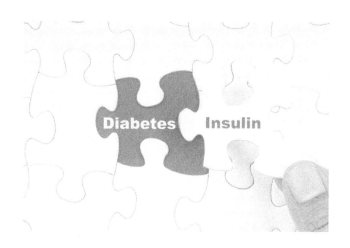

UNDERSTANDING TYPE 2 DIABETES: ITS IMPACT AND MANAGEMENT

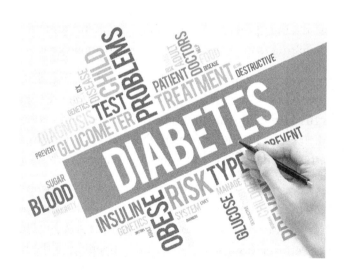

A BRIEF OVERVIEW OF DIABETES HISTORY

Diabetes is a health issue where the body has trouble managing sugar levels in the blood. The first clue about diabetes came from noticing that people with the condition had sweet-tasting pee. This was spotted thousands of years ago by ancient civilizations like the Egyptians, Indians, Chinese, and Greeks.

In the 1600s, an English doctor named Thomas Willis came up with the name "diabetes mellitus" for this problem. But it wasn't until the 1800s that people really started to figure out what was going on with diabetes.

The big breakthrough came in the early 1900s, when two Canadian scientists, Frederick Banting, and Charles Best, discovered a hormone called insulin. Insulin is like a key that aids sugar in getting from your blood into your cells, where it can be used for energy. People with a type of diabetes called type 1 don't have enough insulin, so this discovery led to a treatment that saved many lives.

Later, researchers found out there are different types of diabetes. The most prevalent form is type 2 diabetes, characterized by reduced sensitivity of the body's cells to insulin and insufficient insulin production by the pancreas. Other types include gestational diabetes, occurring during pregnancy in some women, and monogenic diabetes, resulting from genetic alterations in a single gene.

Since then, there have been many advances in handling diabetes. For example, we now have devices that can check blood sugar levels, machines that can deliver insulin (insulin pumps), and better versions of insulin. It's also been confirmed that eating a healthy diet and staying active can make a big difference in managing diabetes.

In recent years, though, we've seen more and more people getting type 2 diabetes around the world. This is mainly because people are moving less, eating less healthy food, and gaining weight. This has led to increased efforts to stop diabetes from happening in the first place, catch it early when it does happen, and manage it effectively.

Nowadays, people with diabetes can manage the condition pretty well. They use medication, change their lifestyle, monitor their condition regularly, and get support and education. Plus, scientists are constantly researching to develop better ways to treat diabetes, stop it from happening, and learn more about it.

In the last few years, there's been a promising development in type 2 diabetes management. Scientists have found that, with advanced eating patterns changes combined with weight loss, T2D can be reversed.

BLOOD SUGAR REGULATION: THE BALANCE IN HEALTHY PEOPLE AND THE DISRUPTION IN TYPE 2 DIABETES

In a healthy body, blood sugar regulation is a finely tuned process. When you eat, your body breaks down a part of food into glucose, or sugar, your body's primary energy source. This increase in blood sugar prompts your pancreas to produce a hormone called insulin. Insulin helps your cells take in the glucose they need for energy. If there's too much glucose, your body stores it in the liver in the form of glycogen, which is how the body keeps a reserve of energy.

Between meals or when you're fasting, when there's no new glucose coming in, your body needs to use its stored energy. That's when the pancreas releases another hormone called glucagon. Glucagon signals your liver to convert its stored glycogen back into glucose and then releases it into the blood. This keeps your blood sugar levels stable.

However, in type 2 diabetes, this process doesn't work as it should. The body's cells become resistant to insulin, which means they can't take in glucose effectively, even though insulin is present. This is like having a locked door with a key that no longer fits. At the same time, the liver continues to produce and release glucose, despite the presence of insulin, which normally signals it to stop. This is similar to a dam releasing water even when it's not needed.

Additionally, glucagon, which should only release stored glucose when needed, doesn't respond to high glucose levels in the blood and continues to release glucose from the liver, causing a surplus. This leads to a condition known as hyperglycemia, or high blood sugar.

In addition, another hormone called amylin, which usually helps to stabilize blood glucose levels after meals, can start to form clumps in the islets of Langerhans. These islets are clusters of specialized cells within the pancreas that include beta cells responsible for insulin production. This leads to an even greater problem with insulin.

All these disruptions in type 2 diabetes cause persistently high blood sugar levels, leading to serious health complications if not effectively managed. Managing type 2 diabetes often involves restoring the normal functioning of blood sugar regulation. This typically involves taking medication, changing diet and exercise habits, regularly monitoring blood sugar levels, and working closely with healthcare professionals.

INSULIN RESISTANCE: THE ONSET STAGE OF TYPE 2 DIABETES

Insulin resistance is like the starting point of type 2 diabetes. When we eat, our body turns the food into glucose, or sugar, which our cells use for energy. Insulin, a hormone made by the beta-cells in the pancreas, helps this glucose get into the cells. But in insulin resistance, the cells start to ignore insulin's signal. It's like insulin is a key, but the lock on the cells is jammed. So, even though there's plenty of insulin around, the glucose can't get into the cells and stays in the blood.

The liver, which also plays a role in managing glucose, gets confused by this. Usually, insulin tells the liver to stop releasing stored glucose into the blood, but in insulin resistance, the liver doesn't get this signal right and keeps releasing glucose. So, there's even more glucose in the blood.

Things get worse because fat cells in people with insulin resistance can release more fatty acids into the blood. These fatty acids can build up in the liver and muscles, worsening insulin resistance.

Over time, the pancreas tries to fix the problem by making more insulin. This leads to too much insulin in the blood, a situation called hyperinsulinemia. But eventually, the pancreas can't keep up with this, and it's unable to make enough insulin. This is when type 2 diabetes can develop.

This journey toward type 2 diabetes usually goes through a few stages:

1. Insulin Resistance: As we just talked about, this is where the cells start to ignore insulin's signal.
2. Compensatory Hyperinsulinemia: In response, the pancreas tries to fix the problem by making more insulin. Blood sugar levels might be normal or a bit high at this stage.
3. Prediabetes: Over time, the pancreas struggles and can't produce enough insulin to stabilize blood sugar within the normal range. Prediabetes is then marked by blood glucose levels above normal but not high enough.
4. Type 2 Diabetes: If the pancreas continues to struggle, it won't be able to make enough insulin, and blood sugar levels go up even more. This is when type 2 diabetes is diagnosed.

The good news is we can often stop this journey towards type 2 diabetes or even reverse it through a Reverse Type 2 Diabetes Diet which helps the body to respond better to insulin.

THE DIAGNOSIS OF TYPE 2 DIABETES

The diagnosis of type 2 diabetes involves measuring blood sugar levels in several ways:

- Fasting blood sugar test: A blood sugar level equal to or exceeding 126 milligrams per deciliter (mg/dL) after not eating or drinking anything except water for at least eight hours indicates diabetes.
- HbA1c test: The results of this blood test reflect your average blood sugar level over the course of the past two to three months. An HbA1c level of 6.5% or higher is considered diabetes.
- Oral glucose tolerance test: A blood sugar level of 200 mg/dL

or above, measured two hours after consuming a sugary solution, can be indicative of diabetes.

Type 2 diabetes can occur due to various factors, including genetics, lifestyle, and environment, but being overweight significantly raises the risk. Managing type 2 diabetes involves:

- Adopting healthier eating habits.
- Incorporating regular exercise.
- Possibly taking medication or insulin to keep blood sugar levels in check.

SYMPTOMS OF TYPE 2 DIABETES

Type 2 diabetes often develops gradually and might not present noticeable symptoms in its early stages. It is common for individuals to live with undiagnosed type 2 diabetes for years. However, noticeable symptoms occur once the blood sugar levels become excessively high. These include:

- Frequent urination and increased thirst: The body attempts to rid itself of excess sugar through urination, leading to dehydration and increased thirst.
- Constant hunger: Lack of sufficient energy from sugar can leave you feeling continuously hungry.
- Unexplained weight loss: The body may start using alternative energy sources like fat, leading to weight loss.
- Fatigue: Insufficient sugar in your cells can constantly tire you.
- Blurred vision: High blood sugar can affect the eyes, causing blurry vision.
- Slow-healing sores or frequent infections: High blood sugar can affect your body's healing process and immunity.
- Darkened skin patches: Areas like the armpits and neck may develop dark patches, often an early sign of insulin resistance.

COMPLICATIONS OF DIABETES

When you have too much sugar in your blood from poorly controlled diabetes, it can cause trouble in different parts of your leading to long-term and devastating complications.

Here's a simple breakdown of how diabetes can affect your body:

- **Blood Vessels and Heart**: When diabetes isn't well managed, sugar builds up in your bloodstream. This can lead to the blood vessels becoming less flexible and narrow, making it difficult for blood to flow properly. The result can be heart-related issues such as high blood pressure, heart disease, and stroke.
- **Nerves**: High blood sugar levels can harm the nerves throughout your body, a condition known as neuropathy. This might cause symptoms like numbness or tingling in your hands or feet, and even pain and weakness in different parts of your body.
- **Kidneys**: Diabetes can also damage your kidneys, which filter waste from your blood. Over time, this damage can get worse, leading to serious kidney problems that might require dialysis or a kidney transplant.
- **Immune System**: High blood sugar can cause inflammation that lasts for a long time, making it harder for your body to fight off infections. This is why people with diabetes may be more predisposed to bacterial, viral, and fungal infections.
- **Bones and Joints**: Diabetes can increase your chances of having bone and joint problems. These can range from a condition known as frozen shoulder, where the movements of your shoulder become limited, to osteoporosis, which weakens your bones and makes them more prone to fractures.
- **Eyes**: Elevated blood sugar levels have the potential to harm the tiny blood vessels in the eyes, resulting in conditions that can significantly impair vision or potentially lead to blindness.

- **Feet**: Damage to your nerves can affect your feet, reducing your ability to feel pain or discomfort. As a result, you may not notice a foot injury, leading to serious complications such as ulcers, infections, and, in severe cases, the necessity of amputation.
- **Teeth and Gums**: Diabetes can lead to problems with your teeth and gums. High blood sugar can result in more plaque on your teeth, resulting in cavities, gum disease, and various other dental problems.

Remember, managing your blood sugar levels effectively is the key to preventing these complications. Regular check-ups can also help to identify and treat any problems early.

UNPACKING THE SCIENCE: THE GI-GL DIET, REVERSING TYPE 2 DIABETES, AND THE TWIN CYCLE HYPOTHESIS

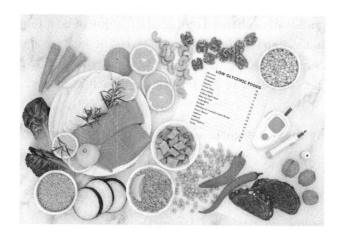

Managing Type 2 diabetes effectively calls for a well-rounded understanding of the scientific principles that shape our dietary choices. With a goal to design a Reverse Type 2 Diabetes Diet that addresses all key facets of a diabetes-reversing, health-promoting diet, we've applied the MECE (Mutually Exclusive, Collectively Exhaustive) framework. This method ensures that:

1. Every component of the diet serves a unique function, signifying that they are mutually exclusive.

2. The diet includes all the essentials for a comprehensive and balanced diet, thus being collectively exhaustive.

By satisfying these conditions, Reverse Type 2 Diabetes Diet stands as a holistic and potent dietary strategy for the reversal of Type 2 diabetes and effective weight management.

UNDERSTANDING THE GLYCEMIC INDEX AND GLYCEMIC LOAD

Reverse Type 2 Diabetes Diet relies heavily on the concepts of Glycemic Index (GI) and Glycemic Load (GL). Introduced by Dr. David Jenkins and his team at the University of Toronto in 1981, the GI has significantly enhanced our understanding of how foods rich in carbohydrates impact blood glucose levels. It assigns a numerical score between 0 and 100 to foods, indicating how quickly they raise blood sugar compared to a reference food such as glucose or white bread.

To simplify, the GI categorizes foods into three main groups:

• Low glycemic index foods: GI less than 55

• Medium glycemic index foods: GI between 56 and 69

• High glycemic index foods: GI more than 70

Initially, the GI focused on promoting the consumption of low-GI foods, moderate intake of medium-GI foods, and avoidance of high-GI foods. However, this approach had a significant drawback as it overlooked the importance of portion sizes. For example, consuming large quantities of low-GI foods, such as skim milk with a relatively high sugar content per serving (24.9g of total sugars per 16 oz), could still lead to elevated blood glucose levels. Moreover, focusing solely on the GI could promote the consumption of potentially unhealthy low-GI foods and overlook the importance of a balanced diet.

Refining the Glycemic Index with Glycemic Load

To rectify these shortcomings of the GI, Harvard University researchers introduced the concept of Glycemic Load (GL). This improved system considers both the quality and the quantity of carbohydrates in a specific food portion, rendering a more holistic and practical measure of its influence on blood sugar levels. In the GL system, 1 GL unit signifies the effect of consuming 1 gram of pure glucose.

Foods are categorized based on their Glycemic Load as:

• Low GL: 10 or less

• Medium GL: 11 to 19

• High GL: 20 or more

The Glycemic Load (GL) plays a pivotal role in the Reverse Type 2 Diabetes Diet. It considers both the Glycemic Index and the quantity of carbohydrates consumed in a single serving when assessing its effect on blood sugar levels. This approach, besides emphasizing carbohydrate quality, underscores the importance of portion control and calorie consciousness.

For instance, while watermelon has a high Glycemic Index (GI), its overall Glycemic Load is low due to the modest amount of carbohydrates in a serving. A serving of watermelon, roughly 1 cup (152g), only contains 11 grams of carbohydrates, resulting in a lower Glycemic Load despite a high GI.

Conversely, parsnips, despite being a low GI food, have a higher carbohydrate content. A serving of cooked parsnip, about 1 cup (215g), contains 35 grams of carbohydrates. This relatively high carbohydrate content results in a higher Glycemic Load compared to watermelon, despite watermelon's higher GI.

THE TWIN CYCLE HYPOTHESIS AND ITS IMPACT ON REVERSING TYPE 2 DIABETES THROUGH FAT ACCUMULATION CONTROL

The Twin Cycle Hypothesis, proposed by Prof. Roy Taylor and his team at Newcastle University, UK, provides valuable insights into the development and treatment of Type 2 diabetes. According to this hypothesis, the disease is initiated by two interconnected cycles: the accumulation of fat in the liver and the accumulation of fat in the pancreas.

The first cycle involves the liver. When an individual consumes more calories than their body needs, the excess energy is stored as fat in the liver. This accumulation of fat impairs the liver's ability to respond to insulin and regulate glucose production, leading to elevated blood sugar levels. Consequently, the pancreas is prompted to increase its production of insulin in order to counterbalance the insulin resistance.

The second cycle involves the pancreas. The increased production of insulin, in response to high blood sugar levels, contributes to the accumulation of fat in the pancreas. This fat accumulation hampers the function of beta cells, which are responsible for producing insulin. As the beta cell function declines, insulin resistance worsens, creating a vicious cycle that eventually leads to the development of Type 2 diabetes.

The significance of the Twin Cycle Hypothesis lies in its implications for the treatment of Type 2 diabetes. If the accumulation of fat in the liver and pancreas is the underlying cause of the disease, then reversing this fat accumulation could potentially reverse the condition itself. Studies have shown that implementing a calorie-restricted diet can effectively decrease the fat content in the liver and pancreas, leading to a restoration of normal insulin production and function.

This understanding marks a paradigm shift in the approach to managing Type 2 diabetes. Rather than solely focusing on symptom management, efforts are directed towards addressing the root cause of the disease. By targeting the fat accumulation in the liver and pancreas, it becomes possible to develop highly effective strategies for preventing and reversing Type 2 diabetes.

INTEGRATING DIETARY STRATEGIES BASED ON TWIN CYCLE HYPOTHESIS FOR EFFECTIVE T2D REVERSAL

In the context of reversing T2D according to the Twin Cycle Hypothesis, the roles of the Glycemic Index (GI), Glycemic Load (GL), and Mediterranean Diet (MedDiet) are particularly significant. By incorporating these dietary approaches, we can address the fat accumulation in the liver and pancreas, which is considered a fundamental factor in the development of Type 2 diabetes.

The GL-focused diet promotes the intake of foods that gradually and consistently release glucose into the bloodstream, thereby curbing excessive insulin response. The aim of this approach is to deter abrupt surges in blood sugar and insulin levels post-meal, which could aid in preventing undue fat deposition in the liver and pancreas. These organs' excessive fat accumulation is posited as a crucial contributor to Type 2 diabetes development, as per the Twin Cycle Hypothesis.

The Mediterranean Diet (MedDiet), renowned for its focus on fruits, vegetables, whole grains, lean proteins, olive oil and healthy fats has been linked to enhanced insulin sensitivity and a decreased likelihood of developing Type 2 diabetes. This diet's nutrient-rich, fiber-packed, and anti-inflammatory properties align with the objective of reducing fat accumulation in the liver and pancreas, potentially reversing the twin cycles associated with the disease.

By merging the principles of the Glycemic Load diet and the Mediterranean Diet, we can forge an effective dietary strategy for naturally reversing Type 2 diabetes, as postulated by the Twin Cycle Hypothesis. This holistic and root cause-focused method has the potential to address this widespread metabolic disorder on a global scale. The significant potential of this scientifically endorsed dietary approach signifies a critical shift in our strategies for managing Type 2 diabetes, potentially ushering in a new era of proactive and effective disease management.

WEIGHT MANAGEMENT: A KEY LEVER IN THE TWIN CYCLE HYPOTHESIS FOR REVERSING TYPE 2 DIABETES

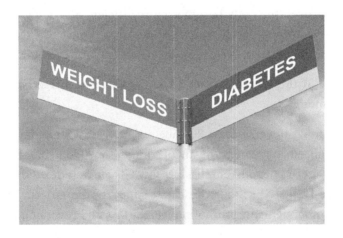

Weight management is at the heart of reversing Type 2 diabetes, as articulated in the Twin Cycle Hypothesis. This theory highlights strategic weight loss to optimize how your body uses glucose and responds to insulin.

Understanding the Role of Weight Management in the Twin Cycle Hypothesis:

The Twin Cycle Hypothesis proposes that Type 2 diabetes emerges from a cycle of excess fat accumulation in the liver and pancreas, often precipitated by chronic overeating. This leads to the onset of insulin resistance and compromised insulin production, ultimately resulting in high blood glucose levels. Yet, strategic weight management can interrupt and reverse this detrimental cycle. When weight management effectively reduces body fat, several beneficial changes follow. Firstly, with diminished fat content, liver function improves, decreasing excessive glucose production, thereby helping maintain balanced blood sugar levels. Secondly, when the fat stored in the pancreas is reduced, the function of beta cells - responsible for insulin production - improves. Consequently, the production and secretion of insulin can be restored to normal levels.

Enhancing insulin sensitivity is a crucial weight management goal in reversing Type 2 diabetes. As body fat decreases and insulin sensitivity improves, the body becomes more efficient at using glucose for energy, resulting in better control of blood sugar levels. This disruption of the detrimental cycle may ultimately lead to reversing T2D.

The Role of the Reverse Type 2 Diabetes Diet in Effective Weight Management:

Implementing Reverse Type 2 Diabetes Diet is instrumental in effective weight management. It incorporates key elements from the Mediterranean Diet and emphasizes low Glycemic Index (GI) and low Glycemic Load (GL) foods. Research supports the efficacy of these dietary components in promoting weight loss and reversing diabetes. For example, the Mediterranean diet has been shown to facilitate significant weight loss, improve blood sugar control, and enhance insulin sensitivity in individuals with Type 2 diabetes. Similarly, a low GI diet has successfully reduced body weight and improved glycemic control in patients with Type 2 diabetes.

Caloric Deficit and its Impact on Weight Loss:

Creating a caloric deficit is essential to weight management and plays a significant role in reversing Type 2 diabetes. A caloric deficit occurs when the energy derived from food intake is less than the energy the body expends. This energy imbalance prompts the body to utilize stored fat reserves for energy, resulting in the process of weight loss.

When a caloric deficit is sustained over time, the body taps into its fat reserves to meet its energy needs. This reduces overall body fat, including the excess fat stored in the liver and pancreas. As body fat decreases, insulin sensitivity often improves, paving the way for better glucose metabolism and blood sugar control.

Amplifying Insulin Sensitivity:

Insulin sensitivity measures how responsive our body's cells are to insulin. In people with Type 2 diabetes, insulin sensitivity is usually reduced, leading to higher blood sugar levels because our cells can't efficiently take in and use glucose. But weight management, which includes creating a caloric deficit and physical activity, can markedly improve insulin sensitivity.

As body fat decreases, particularly in the liver and pancreas, our cells become more receptive to insulin. This allows cells to use glucose more efficiently, reducing blood sugar levels. With enhanced insulin sensitivity, our body can regulate blood sugar levels more effectively and reduce the insulin resistance seen in Type 2 diabetes.

The Impact of Weight Loss on Hormonal Regulation:

Weight loss significantly affects the hormones that control blood sugar levels. Fat cells produce and release various hormones involved in glucose metabolism. When we lose weight and our fat cells decrease in size, this positively affects the balance of these hormones.

Adiponectin is one hormone affected by weight loss. It improves insulin sensitivity and helps break down fatty acids, leading to better fat metabolism. Losing weight has been found to increase levels of adiponectin, which aids in improving insulin function and controlling blood sugar levels.

Leptin, another hormone, is also affected by weight loss. Leptin helps regulate our appetite and energy balance. When we lose weight, leptin levels decrease, which may help curb our appetite and prevent overeating. This supports weight loss efforts and helps control blood sugar levels.

Additionally, weight loss has been associated with lower inflammation markers, such as C-reactive protein (CRP). Less inflammation in the body can improve insulin sensitivity and overall metabolic health.

In conclusion, weight loss achieved through managing weight and creating a caloric deficit can positively impact hormone regulation. This leads to improved insulin sensitivity, better glucose metabolism, and improved blood sugar control.

UNVEILING THE CORE PRINCIPLES OF THE MEDITERRANEAN DIET

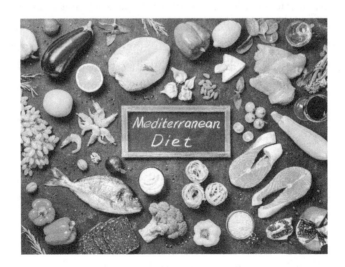

Reverse Type 2 Diabetes Diet integrates key aspects of the Mediterranean diet (MedDiet), improving upon its limitations to create a robust dietary approach to managing and reversing T2D. This innovative diet not only incorporates but also enhances MedDiet's principles, establishing a balanced and healthful eating regimen specifically targeted at T2D management.

One of the core strengths of the Reverse Type 2 Diabetes Diet lies in its embrace of MedDiet's emphasis on plant-based foods, especially those containing glucagon-like peptide agonists. These foods play a crucial role in blood sugar regulation and diabetes control. Furthermore, Reverse Type 2 Diabetes Diet includes foods high in anti-inflammatory and antioxidant properties, which help mitigate the inflammation typically seen in T2D patients.

Reverse Type 2 Diabetes Diet also adopts and enhances MedDiet's focus on the consumption of heart-healthy fats and omega-3 fatty acids. Foods rich in these nutrients not only increase satiety but also enhance insulin efficiency, both vital for weight management and T2D control. Alongside this, Reverse Type 2 Diabetes Diet recommends reducing the intake of red meat and sweets, a principle that aligns with MedDiet. This guideline encourages the consumption of leaner protein sources, helping maintain steady blood sugar levels, decrease overall caloric intake, and facilitate weight loss.

Promoting nutrient-dense eating is another fundamental principle Reverse Type 2 Diabetes Diet adopts from MedDiet. This principle encourages the consumption of foods packed with nutrients over foods abundant in calories but scant in nutrients - the so-called "empty calories." This principle complements the Glycemic Index-Glycemic Load (GI-GL) concepts.

Fruits, vegetables, olive oil, and nuts - foods typical of MedDiet - are rich in anti-inflammatory and antioxidant compounds. Reverse Type 2 Diabetes Diet incorporates these nutrient-dense foods, provided they comply with the low GL, sodium, phosphorus, and potassium guidelines set out in the 2020-2025 Dietary Guidelines. These compounds are crucial for people with T2D as they help to alleviate the heightened inflammation and oxidative stress often accompanying the disease, thereby aiding in better diabetes management.

The gut microbiota-friendly aspect of the MedDiet is a central principle Reverse Type 2 Diabetes Diet has adopted. This principle is essential as a healthier gut microbiota can positively influence how our body processes glucose and uses insulin, making diabetes management more effective. Moreover, the gut microbiota has been linked to the emergence of obesity, metabolic syndrome, and the onset of type 2 diabetes through decreased glucose tolerance and insulin resistance. Numerous studies have demonstrated a significant association between changes in the composition profile of gut microbiota and the development of diabetes.

Lastly, another beneficial feature of the Mediterranean diet adopted by Reverse Type 2 Diabetes Diet is the use of foods containing glucagon-like peptide agonist compounds. These compounds regulate blood sugar levels by promoting insulin release and reducing glucagon secretion - crucial factors for managing T2D.

The integration of these MedDiet principles contributes to the potential benefits of the Reverse Type 2 Diabetes Diet in maintaining stable glucose levels, promoting weight loss, decreasing fat mass, especially around the pancreas and liver, and reducing abdominal fat.

However, while adopting the best MedDiet principles, Reverse Type 2 Diabetes Diet also addresses its shortcomings. For example, it counteracts potential weight gain from consuming high amounts of fat (such as in olive oil and nuts), ensures sufficient iron intake, prevents calcium loss by recommending adequate dairy products, and also considers accessibility and cost of certain Mediterranean foods.

By incorporating the most compelling aspects of the Mediterranean diet and rectifying its limitations, Reverse Type 2 Diabetes Diet paves the way for better blood sugar control, improved insulin sensitivity, and effective weight loss. These principles work synergistically to manage and potentially reverse T2D, providing a complete strategy for optimal health.

EMBRACING THE 2020-2025 DIETARY GUIDELINES AND THEIR IMPORTANCE IN THE TYPE 2 DIABETES REVERSAL DIET

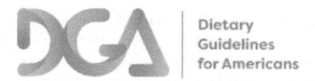

The 2020-2025 Dietary Guidelines for Americans (DGAs) provide evidence-based recommendations for maintaining health and reducing the risk of chronic diseases through nutrition. These guidelines are highly relevant to Reverse Type 2 Diabetes Diet as they complement and enhance its fundamental principles. Let's explore how this symbiosis unfolds and its importance in managing type 2 diabetes (T2D).

Adherence to Nutritional Needs:

The DGAs emphasize that all food and beverage choices matter and contribute to health. The guidelines propose various dietary patterns that meet nutritional needs, decrease the risk of chronic diseases, and promote overall health. Reverse Type 2 Diabetes Diet aligns with this, focusing on nutrient-dense foods, balanced meals, and limiting empty calories, thereby ensuring individuals with T2D meet their nutritional needs while managing blood sugar levels.

Focus on Dietary Patterns:

Both the DGAs and Reverse Type 2 Diabetes Diet prioritize overall dietary patterns over individual nutrients. The DGAs acknowledge that nutrient needs should be met primarily from foods, with each food group providing a variety of essential nutrients. The Mediterranean principles within Reverse Type 2 Diabetes Diet are an excellent example of this focus, emphasizing a variety of nutrient-dense foods and healthy dietary patterns.

Importance of Personalization:

The DGAs underscore that dietary preferences, cultural traditions, and budgetary considerations are important in personalizing dietary guidelines, making them more achievable and sustainable. Reverse Type 2 Diabetes Diet shares this approach, understanding that successful diabetes management and reversal require a diet that individuals can maintain and enjoy in the long run.

Reduction in Added Sugars and Saturated Fats:

The DGAs recommend limiting foods and beverages higher in added sugars and saturated fats. This aligns with Reverse Type 2 Diabetes Diet's principle of limiting sweets and red meat, often high in these components. This focus not only aids in managing blood sugar levels but also supports heart health - an important consideration for individuals with T2D who are at a higher risk of cardiovascular diseases.

Encouragement of Physical Activity:

While not a dietary principle per se, the DGAs recognize the critical role of regular physical activity in supporting health and preventing chronic diseases. Regular exercise can significantly benefit individuals with T2D by improving insulin sensitivity, aiding weight management, and promoting overall health.

In conclusion, the 2020-2025 Dietary Guidelines for Americans align well with the principles of the Reverse Type 2 Diabetes Diet, reinforcing its efficacy. Embracing these guidelines can complement the efforts towards reversing T2D, promoting weight loss, and achieving overall wellness. The principles offer a practical, evidence-based framework that can enhance the management and potential reversal of T2D, making them an integral part of a comprehensive dietary strategy.

THE 17 KEY PRINCIPLES OF THE TYPE 2 DIABETES REVERSAL DIET

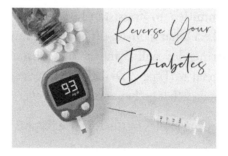

The principles of the Reverse Type 2 Diabetes Diet are highly beneficial because they provide clear and practical guidelines that, with consistent practice, can become ingrained habits. These principles are designed to be adaptable and realistic, making it easier for individuals to sustain them over the long term. As these principles become habits, they require less effort to maintain, ensuring that the dietary changes are sustainable.

Importantly, these principles are not overly restrictive or complicated. They align harmoniously with various healthy dietary patterns, such as the Mediterranean Diet and the recommendations of the 2020-

2025 Dietary Guidelines for Americans. As these principles become habitual, you are more likely to consistently make better decisions, leading to improved weight management, heightened insulin sensitivity, and better adherence to Reverse Type 2 Diabetes Diet.

One crucial point to remember is that habits play a pivotal role in the success of this diet. Reverse Type 2 Diabetes Diet isn't a temporary fix - it's a lifelong commitment designed to prevent the re-accumulation of fat in the pancreas and liver, as explained by the Twin Cycle Hypothesis. The criteria for reversal emphasize that remission is achieved when there is a sustained reduction of HbA1c levels to below 6.5% for at least three months, either occurring spontaneously or as a result of an intervention, without the need for regular glucose-lowering medications.

Therefore, comprehending and implementing these principles is vital. You must be committed to consistently applying them. While this might not seem like a binary, on-or-off approach initially, consistently applying these principles will bring about substantial benefits and speed up the reversal of Type 2 Diabetes. Moreover, these principles will deliver advantages that go beyond merely reversing diabetes:

Here are the 17 key principles of the Reverse Type 2 Diabetes Diet:

1. Embrace Low-Glycemic Load Foods: Prioritize foods with a low glycemic load to effectively manage blood sugar levels.

2. Emphasis on Nutrient Density: Focus on consuming nutrient-dense foods - those high in vitamins, minerals, and other essential nutrients but low in calories to promote overall health and assist in weight management.

3. Limited Intake of Added Sugars and Sweets: Regulate blood glucose levels and decrease overall calorie consumption by minimizing the consumption of foods that are rich in added sugars and sweets.

4. Reduced Consumption of Saturated Fats and Eliminate Trans Fats: Restrict the consumption of trans fats and unhealthy saturated, as

they can have detrimental effects on both heart health and insulin sensitivity. It is recommended to strive for a dietary pattern where saturated fat contributes to approximately 5% to 6% of total calorie intake. (American Heart Association)

5. Choose Healthy Fats and Focus on Heart-Healthy Fats: Opt for foods rich in mono and polyunsaturated fats, such as avocados, nuts, seeds, and olive oil, to support heart health and enhance feelings of satiety.

6. Promotion of Omega-3 Fatty Acids: Enhance insulin sensitivity and mitigate inflammation by incorporating a regular consumption of omega-3-rich foods, such as fatty fish, flaxseeds, and walnuts, into your diet.

7. Stay Active and Regular Physical Activity: Consistent physical activity supports weight management, enhances insulin sensitivity, and improves cardiovascular health.

8. Emphasis on Dietary Patterns: Stress the importance of overall dietary patterns rather than focusing on individual nutrients or foods. This approach promotes a variety of nutrient-rich foods.

9. Attention to Gut Health: Promote foods that support a healthy gut microbiome, such as those high in dietary fiber.

10. Inclusion of Anti-Inflammatory and Antioxidant Foods: Regularly consume foods rich in anti-inflammatory and antioxidant compounds, such as fruits, vegetables, and nuts.

11. Encouragement of Personalization and Recognize Personalization: Acknowledge that food preferences, cultural traditions, and budgetary considerations should be considered when planning a diet. This ensures the dietary plan is enjoyable, sustainable, and effective.

12. Inclusion of Glucagon-Like Peptide Agonist Compounds: Include foods rich in glucagon-like peptide agonist compounds, such as legumes and olive oil, to help regulate blood sugar levels.

13. Incorporate Balanced Protein Intake: Prioritize lean protein sources to maintain muscle mass and keep you feeling satisfied.

14. Stay Hydrated: Drinking sufficient water is crucial for overall health and can aid in blood sugar regulation.

15. Incorporate Polyphenol and Flavonoid-Rich Foods: Consume foods rich in these antioxidants to help combat oxidative stress, a key factor in diabetes.

16. Regular Health Check-Ups: Ensure regular health monitoring to keep track of progress and make necessary adjustments.

17. Embrace a Mediterranean-Inspired Diet: With its focus on fruits, vegetables, whole grains, lean proteins, and healthy fats, MedDiet presents a valuable dietary model that can help in the management of Type 2 diabetes.

EMPIRICAL EVIDENCE SUPPORTING THE T2D REVERSAL DIET

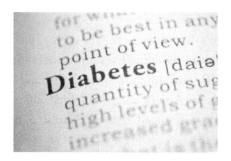

Research and clinical trials illustrate the effectiveness of the Reverse Type 2 Diabetes Diet, underpinned by evidence relating to the Glycemic Index (GI), Glycemic Load (GL), the Mediterranean Diet, and the Twin Cycle Hypothesis in managing Type 2 Diabetes (T2D).

Numerous studies correlate low-GI and low-GL diets with improved blood sugar control in those with T2D. A comprehensive review in the "American Journal of Clinical Nutrition" in 2019 found that low-GI diets notably decrease HbA1c levels, a critical marker of long-term blood sugar control, compared to high-GI diets. Lower HbA1c levels are associated with a decreased risk of diabetes-related complications.

The Mediterranean Diet, central to the Reverse Type 2 Diabetes Diet, shows promise in managing, and potentially reversing T2D. The influential "Prevención con Dieta Mediterránea" (PREDIMED) study revealed that participants following a Mediterranean Diet - supplemented with extra-virgin olive oil or nuts - had a 52% lower risk of developing T2D compared to a low-fat control diet.

At the heart of the Reverse Type 2 Diabetes Diet is Professor Roy Taylor's 'Twin Cycle Hypothesis,' which posits that T2D stems from excess fat in the liver and pancreas, disrupting their normal function. Taylor's groundbreaking research, published in "Diabetes Care" in 2011 and followed by a pivotal study in "The Lancet Diabetes & Endocrinology" in 2016, demonstrated that a low-calorie diet leading to significant weight loss could reduce fat levels in these organs, returning blood glucose levels to normal and potentially inducing T2D remission.

Embracing Taylor's hypothesis, the Reverse Type 2 Diabetes Diet targets weight loss and reducing liver and pancreatic fat. The diet also adheres to low-GI and low-GL principles and incorporates the Dietary Guidelines for Americans, which link nutrient-dense, calorie-conscious eating to a reduced risk of chronic conditions, including T2D complications.

Preliminary research on the Reverse Type 2 Diabetes Diet also indicates its potential in managing T2D. Studies show individuals following this diet see improvements in blood sugar control, weight loss, and reduced reliance on diabetes medication.

While additional long-term, randomized controlled trials are necessary to definitively confirm the effectiveness of the Reverse Type 2 Diabetes Diet, the current body of evidence provides a robust foundation for its potential benefits for individuals with T2D.

RIGHT MACRONUTRIENTS FOR THE TYPE 2 DIABETES REVERSAL DIET

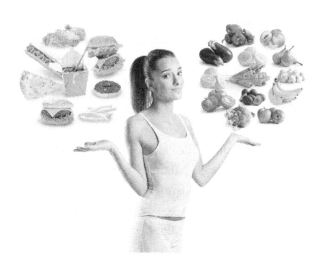

The Western Diet: A Pattern of Concern

The Western diet, common in developed nations, has raised significant health concerns due to its specific attributes. This dietary pattern typically involves high consumption of red and processed meats, sugary desserts, high-fat foods, and refined grains. It also includes frequent intake of high-fat dairy products, sugary drinks, and excessive sodium, while being deficient in essential nutrients found in raw fruits, raw vegetables, whole grains, and lean proteins.

Over time, the energy density of the Western diet has escalated, contributing to numerous health complications. The calorie-dense nature of this diet is intimately tied to the increasing prevalence of conditions like obesity, type 2 diabetes, metabolic disorders, heart disease, and certain cancers, such as colon cancer.

Given these detrimental health impacts associated with the Western diet, a substantial shift towards a healthier, balanced eating pattern becomes crucial. This is where Reverse Type 2 Diabetes Diet steps in. This dietary plan transcends being a temporary fix and becomes a lifestyle change aimed at enhancing overall well-being and battling chronic diseases, particularly type 2 diabetes.

Reverse Type 2 Diabetes Diet encourages distancing from harmful components of the Western diet. It promotes the consumption of raw fruits and vegetables, whole grains, and lean proteins—foods often deficient in a typical Western dietary pattern. This diet also underscores the importance of portion control, regular physical activity, and consistent meal timings.

The objective is to substitute the calorie-dense and unhealthy Western diet with a nutrient-rich, well-balanced eating plan. Gradual adoption of these beneficial dietary adjustments can lead to improved weight management, increased insulin sensitivity, and the effective reversal of type 2 diabetes. By adopting the principles of the Reverse Type 2 Diabetes Diet, individuals can bring about enduring positive changes and enhance their overall health outcomes.

* * *

Understanding Carbohydrates

Carbohydrates play a prominent role in the Western diet, encompassing both complex forms like starch and simple sugars such as sucrose, lactose, and fructose. However, this dietary pattern often falls short in providing adequate microbiota-accessible carbohydrates (MACs), which are crucial for nurturing a healthy gut microbiota community. Insufficient MACs can lead to reduced microbial diversity and a decline in the production of short-chain fatty acids (SCFAs), potentially compromising overall health.

Typically, the Western diet entails a carbohydrate intake ranging from 200-300 grams per day. While carbohydrates serve as a vital energy source for the body, metabolizing into glucose, the high intake can pose challenges for individuals with diabetes in managing blood glucose levels and weight.

The growing prevalence of simple sugars, notably high-fructose corn syrup, in the Western diet raises concerns due to its association with a heightened risk of insulin resistance and type 2 diabetes. Sucrose, primarily found in fruits and vegetables, contributes to approximately 30-35% of carbohydrate intake. Lactose, the dominant sugar in milk and processed foods accounts for around 10-15% of total carbohydrate calories. While fructose naturally occurs in fruits and vegetables, a significant portion is consumed in the form of high-fructose corn syrup.

The process of carbohydrate digestion initiates in the mouth, stomach, and small intestine, where enzymes break down starches and disaccharides into simpler sugars. However, certain carbohydrates, referred to as 'resistant starch,' and undigested sugars bypass this process and proceed to the colon. There, they undergo fermentation by gut bacteria, producing fatty acids that are essential for maintaining gut health and potentially influencing the body's insulin response.

This process can be influenced by the type and preparation of carbohydrates consumed. For instance, raw or minimally processed foods often contain higher amounts of resistant starch compared to highly processed counterparts, providing greater fuel for beneficial gut bacteria.

Carbohydrates are classed as either simple or complex based on their molecular structure. Simple carbohydrates, found in fruits, honey, and sweets, are rapidly metabolized, delivering instant energy but causing abrupt spikes in blood sugar levels. These spikes can potentially contribute to weight gain and difficulties in blood sugar control. In contrast, complex carbohydrates found in whole grains, legumes, and vegetables metabolize slowly, providing a steady and sustainable energy source. They promote blood sugar stability, aid in weight management, and support overall health.

Reverse Type 2 Diabetes Diet draws inspiration from the principles of the Mediterranean diet, as well as the Glycemic Index (GI) and Glycemic Load (GL) framework. This diet recommends that approximately 45-65% of daily caloric intake should come from carbohydrates, with a focus on nutrient-dense, low-GI, and low-GL carbohydrate sources. Additionally, the diet emphasizes the consumption of MACs and high-fiber foods. Diets rich in MACs foster the growth of beneficial gut bacteria and facilitate the production of SCFAs, contributing to enhanced overall health.

Aligned with the 2020-2025 Dietary Guidelines, Reverse Type 2 Diabetes Diet emphasizes the quality of carbohydrates rather than quantity. For effective weight loss and diabetes management, the diet encourages the consumption of foods with a low GI and GL, as well as a high fiber content. Reverse Type 2 Diabetes Diet employs the GL of foods as a guiding compass, determining both the quality and quantity of carbohydrate consumption. Such an approach helps maintain stable blood sugar and insulin levels, aligning with the strategy outlined in the Twin Cycle Hypothesis for breaking the cycle of insulin resistance. By prioritizing high-quality carbohydrates—those that are low-GI, low-GL, and high in fiber—individuals have the potential to improve their metabolic health and reduce the risk of type 2 diabetes.

PROTEINS: ESSENTIAL FOR VITAL FUNCTIONS

Proteins play a multitude of crucial roles in the body, contributing to various bodily functions. They are involved in tissue building and repair, hormone and enzyme production, fluid and acid-base balance maintenance, and support immune function.

For individuals with insulin resistance or a diagnosis of prediabetes, protein deficiency can worsen the condition and hinder the body's ability to regulate glucose levels effectively.

Addressing Protein Deficiency in Diabetes

Proteins are essential macronutrients that form the foundation of numerous bodily functions. These vital compounds contribute to tissue structure and repair, hormone and enzyme production, fluid and acid-base balance, and support immune function.

Proteins are indeed composed of a set of 20 standard amino acids, each with unique properties. These amino acids have the ability to form bonds with each other in a variety of sequences, allowing for an immense diversity of possible protein structures. Each unique sequence of amino acids results in a unique protein with its own structure and function. This diversity is essential for the complex biological processes that sustain life. Among these amino acids, nine are considered essential as the body cannot produce them internally. Hence, they must be obtained through the diet. These essential amino acids, including histidine, isoleucine, leucine, lysine, methionine, phenylalanine, threonine, tryptophan, and valine, play critical roles in protein synthesis, growth, tissue repair, and maintenance. They are also implicated in the production of enzymes, hormones, and neuro-transmitters.

According to the guidance of the American Diabetes Association (ADA), patients with diabetes and early stages of chronic kidney disease should aim for a protein intake of 0.8–1.0 g/kg per day, reducing it to 0.8 g/kg per day in the later stages of kidney disease.

Adequate protein intake plays a crucial role in enhancing the overall health and well-being of individuals with diabetes, as it helps prevent the decline of muscle mass and reduces the likelihood of falls and injuries.

Generally, animal-based protein sources (e.g., meat, poultry, fish, eggs, dairy products) are considered complete protein sources since they typically provide all the essential amino acids necessary for the body. Plant-based proteins, found in legumes, grains, nuts, and seeds, may lack certain essential amino acids individually. However, by incorporating a variety of plant-based proteins into the daily diet, it is possible to obtain all the essential amino acids required.

Meeting the recommended protein intake offers numerous benefits, particularly regarding glycemic control. Adequate protein intake can help lower HbA1c levels, a marker of long-term blood sugar control. Proteins also enhance the insulin response, preventing sudden spikes in blood sugar. Additionally, they aid in hunger control and promote satiety, which can support weight management efforts. Furthermore, research indicates that proteins can lower the glycemic index of a meal, thereby reducing the risk of post-meal blood sugar spikes.

High-quality protein sources include lean meats (e.g., chicken, turkey, fish like salmon and tuna, eggs), dairy products (e.g., Greek yogurt, cottage cheese,) plant-based sources (e.g., chickpeas, quinoa, soy products), and Nuts and seeds (e.g., almonds, walnuts, chia seeds, flax seeds).

The 30-day meal plan provided in the Reverse Type 2 Diabetes Diet is specifically designed to offer an adequate amount of protein, incorporating a balance of both plant and animal sources. This meal plan serves as a practical and straightforward guide for meeting daily protein requirements while aiming to reverse type 2 diabetes.

FATS: ESSENTIAL MACRONUTRIENTS FOR OPTIMAL HEALTH

Fats have a vital role in our diet, fulfilling important functions in cell structure, hormone regulation, and promoting the health of the heart and brain. They serve as a potent source of energy, especially when food intake is limited or during extended periods of physical activity, as the body utilizes stored fats for fuel. Furthermore, fats facilitate the absorption of fat-soluble vitamins A, D, E, and K, thereby enhancing nutrient intake and supporting metabolic processes.

The human diet consists of three main types of fats:

- **Saturated Fats**: Primarily found in animal-based foods and certain plant-based sources, overconsumption of saturated fats is associated with increased LDL ("bad") cholesterol levels, raising the risk of heart disease and other cardiovascular problems. Therefore, it is advisable to limit saturated fat intake.
- **Unsaturated Fats**: Considered healthier than saturated fats, unsaturated fats can be subdivided into monounsaturated and polyunsaturated fats. They help improve blood cholesterol levels and support overall heart health. Foods abundant in unsaturated fats include olive oil, avocados, certain nuts, fatty fish, seeds, and some vegetable oils.
- **Trans Fats**: Artificially formed through hydrogenation to solidify liquid oils and prolong shelf life, trans fats are commonly found in processed and commercially packaged foods. They raise LDL cholesterol levels while lowering HDL ("good") cholesterol levels, posing significant risks to heart health and overall well-being.

The prevalent Western diet, characterized by a high intake of omega-6 fatty acids, saturated fats, and trans fats and a low intake of omega-3 fatty acids, is a cause for concern. This dietary pattern can promote inflammation, insulin resistance, and type 2 diabetes. Moreover, an imbalance between omega-6 and omega-3 fatty acids intake exacerbates inflammation and fosters insulin resistance. It is, therefore, crucial to rectify this imbalance for optimal health.

Recommended Intake and Effects on Diabetes Risk:

Scientific evidence suggests that different types of fats may have varying effects on the risk for type 2 diabetes (T2D). It is important to note that dietary fat does not directly impact blood sugar levels, but consuming a high-fat meal can slow digestion and lower the glycemic index (GI), which mitigates the speed at which blood sugar levels rise after eating.

Furthermore, data from prospective cohort studies indicate that the quality of fats consumed can influence insulin sensitivity and, consequently, the risk of T2D. Diets high in saturated fatty acids (SFAs) have been associated with a raised risk of T2D, while diets rich in polyunsaturated fatty acids (PUFAs) have shown beneficial effects, potentially reducing the risk of diabetes.

Based on these findings, the following are the recommended daily intakes of fats, which can be adjusted according to individual dietary needs and lifestyle:

- **Saturated Fats:** As a general guideline, saturated fats should make up less than 10% of total daily caloric intake due to their potential to increase LDL cholesterol levels and heighten the likelihood of heart disease and T2D.
- **Unsaturated Fats:** These fats, including both monounsaturated and polyunsaturated fats, are healthier alternatives to saturated fats. They should constitute the majority of fat intake, replacing SFAs whenever possible. Specifically, regular inclusion of PUFAs, known for their protective effects against diabetes, is recommended.
- **Trans Fats:** Given their negative health impacts, trans fats should be limited as much as possible. The World Health

Organization recommends a trans fat intake of less than 1% of total energy intake.

In line with these recommendations, a dietary strategy for T2D reversal emphasizes shifting from SFAs to PUFAs while maintaining a balanced and nutrient-rich diet. This dietary modification can significantly enhance insulin sensitivity.

MICRONUTRIENTS, GUT HEALTH, AND LIFESTYLE: THE SUPPORTING PILLARS

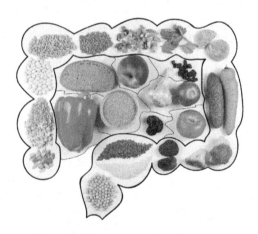

Reverse Type 2 Diabetes Diet is carefully designed to acknowledge the crucial interactions among nutrients, highlighting symbiotic pairs like Vitamin D and Calcium that optimize nutrient absorption and enhance bone strength.

This diet encourages consuming foods rich in Vitamin B12 and Folate due to their synergistic role in cell division and replication, crucial processes for maintaining optimal health. To handle potential adversarial relationships between minerals like zinc and copper, the diet advises a balanced intake to prevent deficiencies or excesses.

While macronutrients are vital for fulfilling our dietary needs, it's equally important to acknowledge the role of micronutrients such as vitamins and minerals. They may not serve as direct energy sources, but they play vital roles in orchestrating critical biological functions like energy synthesis, enzyme activation, and bone health fortification.

Micronutrients are instrumental in enhancing blood glucose control, crucial for individuals managing T2D. Reverse Type 2 Diabetes Diet emphasizes key micronutrients particularly beneficial for managing this condition:

- **Vitamin D:** Adequate levels of Vitamin D have been associated with enhanced insulin sensitivity, which is crucial for breaking the cycle of insulin resistance commonly seen in Type 2 Diabetes.
- **Vitamin K:** Vitamin K is involved in glucose metabolism and has been found to increase insulin sensitivity, potentially aiding in better blood sugar control.
- **Magnesium:** Magnesium plays a role in activating metabolic enzymes and cellular transporters involved in glucose uptake and utilization. Adequate magnesium intake has been associated with improved blood sugar control.
- **Vitamin C:** Vitamin C, due to its antioxidant properties, protects the body against oxidative stress. It also supports the immune system, which is essential for overall health, including diabetes management.
- **B-Vitamins:** B vitamins, including B12 and folate, are involved in energy production, nerve function, and the regulation of homocysteine levels. They are essential for maintaining good health and supporting various biological processes.
- **Chromium:** Chromium is a mineral known for its ability to

improve insulin function and regulate blood sugar levels within the normal range. It has been studied for its potential benefits in glucose control.

- **Zinc:** Zinc plays a crucial role in supporting immune function, facilitating wound healing, and promoting insulin production. Adequate zinc levels may contribute to improved insulin sensitivity and overall metabolic health.
- **Calcium:** Calcium is crucial for bone health, nerve function, and muscle contractions. It works synergistically with vitamin D to enhance nutrient absorption and support bone strength.

* * *

THE ROLE OF GUT HEALTH AND MICROBIOME IN REVERSE TYPE 2 DIABETES DIETT

The role of the gut microbiome in managing type 2 diabetes (T2D) is a rapidly emerging field. The gut microbiome comprises trillions of microorganisms, including bacteria, fungi, and viruses, that inhabit our digestive tract. Studies have shown that imbalances in this community, also known as dysbiosis, may contribute to insulin resistance and T2D.

The mechanisms proposed through which the gut microbiome influences T2D include:

- **Metabolic Functions:** The gut microbiome helps ferment undigested dietary fibers, producing short-chain fatty acids (SCFAs) such as acetate, propionate, and butyrate. These SCFAs play a role in regulating glucose metabolism and insulin sensitivity.
- **Inflammation:** Dysbiosis in the gut microbiome can lead to chronic low-grade inflammation, known to contribute to insulin resistance, a characteristic feature of T2D.
- **Gut Barrier Function:** The gut lining functions as a barrier,

preventing harmful substances from entering the bloodstream. If this barrier is compromised, often referred to as "leaky gut," bacteria and their toxins can leak into the bloodstream, leading to inflammation and metabolic dysfunction.

- **Bile Acid Metabolism:** The gut microbiome contributes to the metabolism of bile acids, which play a role in regulating lipid metabolism, glucose balance, and energy homeostasis. Changes in the gut microbiome can affect these bile acid profiles, potentially impacting metabolic health.
- Given these considerations, dietary modifications that can improve gut health and modulate the gut microbiome composition may be beneficial for T2D management:
- **High-fiber Diet:** A diet high in fiber, especially from diverse plant-based sources, encourages the growth of beneficial bacteria, enhancing the production of SCFAs that can improve insulin sensitivity and decrease inflammation.
- **Probiotics and Prebiotics:** Probiotics (beneficial live bacteria consumed through certain foods or supplements) and prebiotics (non-digestible fibers that act as food for these beneficial bacteria) can help restore a healthy balance in the gut microbiome.
- **Polyphenol-rich Foods:** Polyphenols, found in foods like berries, green tea, and cocoa, possess antioxidant and anti-inflammatory properties. They can modulate the gut microbiome to promote metabolic health.
- **Reduced Intake of Added Sugars and Highly Processed Foods:** Diets high in added sugars and ultra processed foods can disrupt gut health and encourage the growth of harmful bacteria. Reducing these foods can support a healthier gut microbiome.

Incorporating these strategies into Reverse Type 2 Diabetes Diet offers potential benefits in managing this condition by promoting a healthier gut microbiome.

* * *

THE IMPACT OF SLEEP AND STRESS ON LIFESTYLE FACTORS

Recognizing the significance of sleep and stress concerning lifestyle factors is crucial, as they profoundly influence blood sugar control, weight management, and overall well-being. Reverse Type 2 Diabetes Diet considers these non-dietary factors to provide a comprehensive approach. Insufficient sleep and high stress levels can exacerbate insulin resistance. Conversely, ensuring adequate sleep and managing stress levels can enhance the benefits derived from a diet that is low in glycemic glycemic load and adheres to the principles of Mediterranean-style eating.

By addressing sleep and stress as integral components of the Reverse Type 2 Diabetes Diet, individuals can optimize their overall health and improve their ability to manage blood sugar levels. Adequate rest and stress management contribute to better insulin sensitivity and the successful implementation of a diet that minimizes fluctuations in blood sugar levels. This comprehensive approach recognizes the interconnectedness of various lifestyle factors and their impact on the management and reversal of type 2 diabetes, promoting improved health outcomes.

* * *

Understanding the Psychological Aspects of Eating

Understanding How We Think About Eating Managing your diet Recognizing how our thoughts and emotions influence our eating habits is crucial for successfully managing our diet. Reverse Type 2 Diabetes Diet acknowledges that achieving optimal health is not solely about consuming nutritious foods and maintaining balanced meals; it also involves understanding our psychological relationship with food. By identifying the triggers for emotional eating, practicing mindfulness while eating, and gaining insight into our individual eating habits, we can cultivate a healthier and more balanced approach to food. These principles align with the Mediterranean diet, which emphasizes not only the nutritional aspects of food but also the enjoyment of eating.

THE TYPE 2 DIABETES REVERSAL DIET VS OTHER DIETS

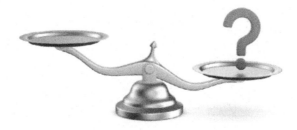

Comparing various dietary approaches clarifies why Reverse Type 2 Diabetes Diet may be the most suitable for those aiming to manage and potentially reverse Type 2 diabetes. Let's see how it fares against other diets:

- **Carb Counting:** Carb Counting: Essential for those on insulin, it helps manage carbohydrate intake and control blood sugar. Reverse Type 2 Diabetes Diet advances this by integrating the Mediterranean and Glycemic Load diets. It offers a holistic approach focusing on both carb quantity and quality, tackles insulin resistance, and promotes weight loss. By blending nutrient-rich Mediterranean foods and considering glycemic load, it ensures well-rounded nutrition and efficient blood sugar management, exceeding the capabilities of mere carb counting. The diet's focus on weight loss also supports diabetes reversal.

- **Mediterranean Diet:** The Mediterranean Diet, famed for promoting heart health, primarily consists of fruits, vegetables, whole grains, fish, lean meats, and olive oil. While this is a healthy approach, it doesn't emphasize portion control, especially for high glycemic index fruits like watermelon, figs, and grapes, which can lead to potential weight gain. Furthermore, it might not provide sufficient iron and calcium. Reverse Type 2 Diabetes Diet builds upon the Mediterranean Diet's principles and the glycemic load concept, but it explicitly addresses these shortcomings. By focusing on portion control and integrating strategies to combat insulin resistance, Reverse Type 2 Diabetes Diet provides a comprehensive approach to ultimately reversing blood sugar levels.

- **Glycemic Load Diet:** while both the Glycemic Load Diet and Reverse Type 2 Diabetes Diet consider the glycemic load of foods, Reverse Type 2 Diabetes Diet offers a broader approach by incorporating the best elements of the Mediterranean Diet and targeting insulin sensitivity and belly fat reduction. This comprehensive approach sets it apart as a more holistic and effective strategy for managing and reversing type 2 diabetes.

- **DASH Diet:** Created to lower high blood pressure, the DASH diet endorses reduced sodium intake and promotes nutrient-rich foods. While it aligns with Reverse Type 2 Diabetes Diet's focus on whole foods, it doesn't emphasize glycemic index or load, crucial aspects of the Reverse Type 2 Diabetes Diet. Additionally, it does not provide strategies to combat insulin resistance and target belly fat loss.

- **Flexitarian Diet:** A fusion of 'flexible' and 'vegetarian,' this diet accentuates plant-based foods but allows occasional meat intake. It shares Reverse Type 2 Diabetes Diet's flexibility and nutrient-dense food focus, but it doesn't specifically target blood glucose level management or directly address insulin resistance or central adiposity reduction.
- **MIND Diet:** A hybrid of the Mediterranean and DASH diets, the MIND diet focuses on foods that benefit brain health. While its principles align with many aspects of the Reverse Type 2 Diabetes Diet, it doesn't specifically address blood glucose regulation and insulin resistance reversal. Reverse Type 2 Diabetes Diet provides a more comprehensive approach, prioritizing glycemic control and directly tackling insulin resistance.
- **Vegetarian Diet:** This diet, rich in vegetables, fruits, and whole grains, overlaps with Reverse Type 2 Diabetes Diet. However, it doesn't focus specifically on glycemic index and load or strategies for reversing insulin resistance. It also may lead to nutritional deficiencies in nutrients found predominantly in animal-based foods.
- **Noom and the New Mayo Clinic Diet:** These weight loss programs incorporate behavioral changes to promote healthier eating and exercise. While they share similarities with Reverse Type 2 Diabetes Diet, they do not provide specific strategies for blood glucose regulation, reversing insulin resistance, and targeting central adiposity.
- **Pescatarian and Flexitarian Diets:** Although these diets incorporate healthy eating principles, they don't specifically target glycemic index, glycemic load, or strategies for reversing T2D. Reverse Type 2 Diabetes Diet, on the other hand, is specifically designed to address all these factors and more. It aims to help individuals manage their blood glucose levels effectively, improve insulin sensitivity, and target weight loss around the abdomen.
- **Ketogenic (Keto) Diet:** The Keto diet may lead to rapid

weight loss and decreased blood sugar levels through a high-fat, low-carb approach. However, it often includes high levels of saturated fats. While there are some parallels with Reverse Type 2 Diabetes Diet, such as an emphasis on controlling blood glucose levels, the Reversal Diet underscores the consumption of healthy fats and advocates for sustainable weight loss and blood sugar control. It also addresses insulin resistance directly, an area not explicitly targeted in the Keto diet.

- **Paleo Diet:** The Paleo diet emphasizes foods that prehistoric humans may have eaten, such as meat, fish, fruits, and vegetables, while excluding processed foods and grains. While it shares Reverse Type 2 Diabetes Diet's emphasis on whole foods, it doesn't specifically address the glycemic index or load nor includes strategies to tackle insulin resistance directly.

- **Vegan Diet:** The Vegan diet eliminates all animal-derived products, focusing on plant-based foods. While it overlaps with Reverse Type 2 Diabetes Diet in its emphasis on plant-based, nutrient-dense foods, it lacks a specific focus on glycemic control and reversing insulin resistance. Additionally, it might lead to deficiencies in nutrients predominantly found in animal-based foods, such as Vitamin B12, unless well-planned.

- **Intermittent Fasting (IF):** Intermittent fasting is a practice that entails alternating between periods of eating and fasting. This approach aligns with Reverse Type 2 Diabetes Diet's emphasis on insulin regulation. However, Reverse Type 2 Diabetes Diet provides a more rounded dietary approach, focusing not just on eating timings but also on the quality of foods, their glycemic load, and lifestyle changes to address insulin resistance and target abdominal fat loss.

- **Whole30 Diet:** The Whole30 diet is a 30-day plan designed to reset your eating habits by cutting out certain food groups, including sugar, grains, legumes, and dairy. While it shares a focus on whole foods with Reverse Type 2 Diabetes Diet, it lacks specific attention to glycemic index and load and does not provide strategies to reverse insulin resistance or target central adiposity. Reverse Type 2 Diabetes Diet, in contrast, takes a more comprehensive, longer-term approach to dietary and lifestyle changes.

PART II
MASTERING MEAL PLANNING FOR THE TYPE 2 DIABETES REVERSAL DIET

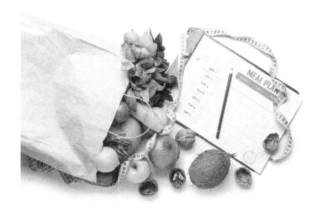

MAPPING YOUR MEAL PLAN FOR THE TYPE 2 DIABETES REVERSAL DIET

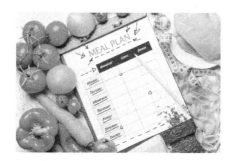

Reverse Type 2 Diabetes Diet's comprehensive meal plan is a calculated strategy that aims to optimize blood glucose control, enhance insulin sensitivity, aid weight loss, and decrease diabetes-related risks. It smartly merges the 17 principles of the Reverse Type 2 Diabetes Diet with beneficial aspects of the Mediterranean and Glycemic Load diets while addressing their limitations to guide food choice.

Reverse Type 2 Diabetes Diet's integrated approach encapsulates healthy nutrition, lifestyle, and well-being factors, ensuring all critical aspects of MedDiet and GI-GL diets for managing and potentially reversing Type 2 diabetes are covered.

By borrowing the health benefits of the Mediterranean and Glycemic Load diets, including better heart health and glycemic control, Reverse Type 2 Diabetes Diet maximizes its effectiveness. It highlights low glycemic load, whole, nutrient-rich foods like fruits, vegetables, whole grains, lean proteins, and healthy fats like olive oil while addressing the blindspots, such as careless fruit consumption that can impact blood sugar and weight gain due to lack of portion control.

Key Features of the Comprehensive Meal Planning Approach:

1. **Glycemic Index and Glycemic Load:** in the Reverse Type 2 Diabetes Diet, a key emphasis is placed on understanding and utilizing foods' glycemic index (GI) and glycemic load (GL). This knowledge not only aids in achieving better blood sugar control and weight loss but also reduces the risk of diabetes-related complications. By providing practical guidance, such as ranking foods based on their GI, GL, serving size, and net carbs, individuals can make informed food choices. This approach fosters improved insulin sensitivity, weight management, and overall health.

2. **Mediterranean Diet Influence:** The meal planning approach draws inspiration from the Mediterranean diet, which emphasizes heart-healthy fats, lean proteins, and a diverse array of fruits, vegetables, and whole grains. This dietary pattern is associated with lower diabetes rates and improved glycemic control.

3. **Weight Management:** Weight loss, achieved through a caloric deficit, is crucial to reversing type 2 diabetes. Managing weight effectively leads to improved blood sugar control and a significantly reduced risk of diabetes-related complications.

4. **Comorbidity Management:** The diet addresses the prevalence of comorbid conditions among individuals with diabetes, such as hypertension and heart disease, by providing dietary recommendations that cater to these conditions. This promotes a holistic approach to managing overall health.

5. **Prevention of Life-threatening Complications:** By managing blood glucose levels through a nutrient-rich diet, the diet significantly reduces the likelihood of severe complications such as kidney disease, nerve damage, heart disease, and stroke.

6. **Personalization and Flexibility:** The diet encourages customization based on individual needs, food preferences, and lifestyle factors. It provides a flexible structure or framework that can be adapted to various situations and requirements.

7. **Integration of Latest Nutritional Guidelines:** The meal planning approach aligns with the 2020-2025 Dietary Guidelines for Americans, emphasizing the consumption of a variety of nutrient-dense foods while limiting added sugars, saturated fats, and sodium intake.

8. **Addressing Psychological Aspects of Eating:** The diet recognizes and addresses emotional eating triggers, the importance of mindful eating, and the development of a healthier relationship with food. It acknowledges the psychological factors that can influence dietary choices.

This approach provides not only a tool for managing diabetes and promoting weight loss but also a sustainable and flexible dietary lifestyle that promotes long-term health and well-being.

CREATING YOUR PERSONALIZED MEAL PLAN

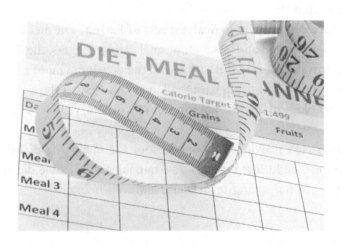

Creating a tailored meal plan is critical for effective diabetes management and weight loss. This plan should reflect your health goals, food preferences, and lifestyle, balancing essential nutrients to support diabetes reversal efforts. Here's how you can personalize a plan:

Define Your Health Goals and Dietary Preferences: Clearly identify your goals, such as weight loss or improved blood glucose control, and consider any dietary restrictions or personal food preferences. Also, consider your daily routine and available meal preparation time.

Embrace the Mediterranean Diet Principles: Ensure your meal plan includes vegetables, fruits, lean proteins, whole grains, and heart-healthy fats like olive oil, all central to the Mediterranean diet.

Incorporate Low GI-GL Foods: Diversify your diet with an assortment of low glycemic index (GI) and glycemic load (GL) foods. Always check their GI and GL values when available. This strategy counters the potential drawbacks of the Mediterranean diet by limiting the intake of high-carbohydrate foods like watermelon, figs, grapes, and dates, which have higher carb content and can potentially impact blood sugar control.

Prioritize Weight Loss: Weight loss is crucial as it plays a significant role in reversing type 2 diabetes. Achieving a caloric deficit is important, and this can be supported by implementing portion control strategies and including low-calorie, nutrient-dense foods.

Integrate the 17 Principles: The 17 principles of the Reverse Type 2 Diabetes Diet provide a comprehensive framework for food choices, meal timing, and nutrient balance.

Regulate Meal Frequency and Timing: Consistent meal times and frequency are significant for blood glucose control and weight management. Regular meals and smaller, more frequent eating can maintain stable blood glucose levels and prevent overeating.

Balance Macronutrients: Regulate your intake of carbohydrates, proteins, and fats for blood glucose control and weight management. Include low-GI carbohydrates, lean proteins, and heart-healthy fats.

Plan for Special Situations: Be prepared for situations like dining out, managing other health conditions, or adjusting plans for physical activity. Research restaurant menus in advance, consult your healthcare team for comorbidity management and adjust meals based on physical activities.

By aligning your meal plan with your unique needs and integrating Mediterranean diet principles and the 17 principles of the Reverse Type 2 Diabetes Diet, you can create a sustainable, effective path towards managing and potentially reversing type 2 diabetes.

CRAFTING YOUR ESSENTIAL SHOPPING LIST FOR THE TYPE 2 DIABETES REVERSAL DIET

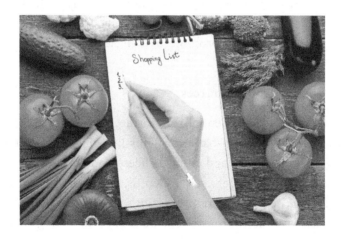

Embarking on a journey towards a balanced and sustainable diet for reversing Type 2 Diabetes might initially seem daunting, especially when navigating through the multitude of options in supermarket aisles. However, with a strategic and well-structured shopping list, healthier choices become accessible, ensuring consistent adherence to the principles of the Reverse Type 2 Diabetes Diet. This aims to equip you with strategies for crafting a shopping list that aligns with your health goals, weight management objectives, and the Mediterranean diet. These strategies will help you make informed choices when selecting foods and create a foundation for your healthy eating habits.

A. Planning Ahead for Success

A well-executed diet begins with thoughtful planning. Create a shopping list before entering the store to resist impulse purchases that might veer you off your dietary objectives. Allocate time each week to strategize meals and snacks that meet your nutritional needs and weight loss goals while aligning with your diabetes reversal efforts. Your shopping list becomes your roadmap to better health.

B. Embracing Whole and Minimally Processed Foods

When constructing your shopping list, focus on fresh, whole, or minimally processed foods that align with Reverse Type 2 Diabetes Diet. Prioritize lean proteins, Low-GI whole grains, fruits, vegetables, and healthy fats, all of which promote overall health and help maintain stable blood sugar levels.

C. Diversifying Protein Sources

Lean proteins play an essential role in the Reverse Type 2 Diabetes Diet. Include both animal-based proteins like chicken breast, turkey, fish, eggs, Greek yogurt, and cottage cheese and plant-based proteins like legumes, tofu, tempeh, seitan, lentils, chickpeas, and edamame. These proteins deliver vital nutrients without excessive unhealthy fats and calories, keeping your meals balanced and supporting your health goals.

D. Prioritizing Low-GL and Fiber-Rich Foods

Strive for a diverse selection of fruits and vegetables with low GL values, such as cherries, plums, peaches, apricots, apples, oranges, pears, and most berries. Fiber-rich foods (e.g., whole grains, legumes, fruits, and vegetables) should also feature prominently on your shopping list as they slow the absorption of carbohydrates, leading to more stable blood sugar levels.

E. Incorporating Healthy Fats

Healthy fats derived from sources such as extra virgin olive oil, avocados, nuts, and seeds play a vital role in the Reverse Type 2 Diabetes Diet. These fats are packed with essential fatty acids, contribute to increased meal satisfaction, and assist in balancing the glycemic index (GI) of your meals.

F. Avoiding Sugary Drinks and Highly Processed Foods

Replace sugary drinks and highly processed foods, which usually have high GI values, with whole foods, water, unsweetened coffee or tea, or sparkling water. These healthier options can prevent rapid blood sugar spikes and potential health issues.

G. Selecting Low-GL Snacks

Keep a variety of healthy, low-GL snacks at hand to satisfy hunger between meals. Snacks like nuts, seeds, and raw veggies with hummus can stabilize blood sugar levels.

H. Navigating the Supermarket

As a general rule, focus your shopping on the store's perimeter, which typically features fresh produce, lean proteins, and dairy products—all perfect for a Reverse Type 2 Diabetes Diet. Also, explore local farmers' markets or ethnic grocery stores for a wider variety of fresh produce and whole grain products.

I. Becoming a Label Detective

When buying packaged foods, scrutinize nutrition labels for added sugars, sodium, and trans fats. Ensure the product fits within the guidelines of the Reverse Type 2 Diabetes Diet. An informed shopper makes healthier choices.

In conclusion, transitioning to Reverse Type 2 Diabetes Diet doesn't have to be complex. A well-thought-out shopping list, coupled with the guidelines outlined above, can streamline your journey toward weight loss, enhanced diabetes control, and a healthier lifestyle.

Always plan your meals, diversify your protein sources, and prioritize whole foods for a healthier and balanced diet.

COOKING TECHNIQUES AND MEAL PREPARATION: MASTERING THE ART

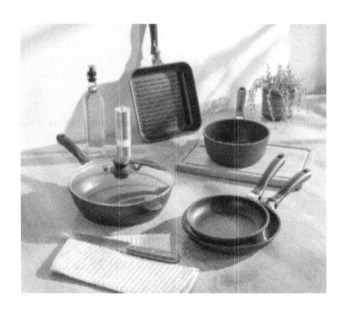

The food we eat and how it's prepared can significantly impact the management and potential reversal of Type 2 Diabetes. According to the twin cycle hypothesis, the reduction of fat stores in the pancreas and liver, which is crucial for reversing Type 2 Diabetes, is directly influenced by our dietary choices and cooking methods. Adhering to

Reverse Type 2 Diabetes Diet principles, optimizing cooking techniques to retain nutritional value, and focusing on reducing the Glycemic Index (GI) and Glycemic Load (GL) of meals are integral aspects of effectively managing and potentially reversing diabetes.

Let's examine the pros and cons of various cooking techniques that align with the principles of the Reverse Type 2 Diabetes Diet and support your efforts in reversing diabetes.

1. BAKING

- **Pros:** Minimal added fat, ideal for preparing lean meats, fish, poultry, vegetables, and whole-grain dishes.
- **Cons:** Can result in the loss of some water-soluble vitamins due to extended cooking times and high temperatures.

2. BROILING

- **Pros:** Creates a flavorful crust while retaining moisture, ideal for lean proteins and vegetables.
- **Cons:** Can produce potentially harmful substances like heterocyclic amines (HCAs) and polycyclic aromatic hydrocarbons (PAHs) when cooking meat at high temperatures.

3. GRILLING

- **Pros:** Imparts a unique, smoky flavor and cooks food quickly with minimal added fat. Ideal for lean meats, fish, vegetables, and fruits.
- **Cons:** Similar to broiling, can produce HCAs and PAHs when cooking meat at high temperatures.

4. POACHING

- **Pros:** Requires no added fat and helps retain nutrients. Perfect for delicate proteins like fish, eggs, and poultry.
- **Cons:** May produce less flavorful dishes than other methods. To enhance the flavor, consider using seasoned poaching liquids.

5. ROASTING

- **Pros:** Cooks food evenly and develops rich flavors, ideal for meats, poultry, and vegetables.
- **Cons:** Can result in losing some nutrients due to extended cooking times and high temperatures.

6. PRESSURE COOKING

- **Pros:** Reduces cooking times and helps retain nutrients, ideal for legumes, whole grains, and tenderizing tough cuts of meat.
- **Cons:** Can be intimidating for some users, and improper use can lead to overcooked or undercooked food.

7. SLOW COOKING

- **Pros:** Requires minimal hands-on time and develops deep, complex flavors. Perfect for soups, stews, and tenderizing tough cuts of meat.
- **Cons:** Can result in losing some nutrients due to extended cooking times and high temperatures.

8. STIR-FRYING OR SAUTÉING

- **Pros:** Cooks food quickly over high heat, helping retain nutrients and develop vibrant flavors. Ideal for vegetables, lean proteins, and whole grains.
- **Cons:** Requires some oil or fat, which can increase the calorie content of a dish. Always use heart-healthy oils in moderation.

9. STEAMING

- **Pros:** Requires no added fat and helps retain nutrients and moisture. Ideal for vegetables, fish, and shellfish.
- **Cons:** Steamed dishes may lack the depth of flavor associated with other cooking methods.

10. NO-COOK

- **Pros:** Helps to conserve the maximum amount of nutrients in food. These recipes often include raw fruits, vegetables, and simple salads.
- **Cons:** No-cook recipes may not be as filling or satisfying as cooked dishes.

* * *

PLANNING AND PREPARING MEALS IN ADVANCE

Proactive meal planning plays a significant role in the Reverse Type 2 Diabetes Diet. By incorporating the following strategies, you can improve blood glucose control, facilitate weight loss, and make substantial strides toward diabetes reversal:

1. **Weekly meal planning:** Design a meal plan for the week ahead that incorporates the principles of the Mediterranean diet and Reverse Type 2 Diabetes Diet. This will involve including an assortment of low-glycemic index (GI) foods, lean sources of protein, healthy fats, and low-GL fruits and vegetables.
2. **Shopping list preparation:** Develop a detailed shopping list based on your meal plan to stay organized and avoid impulse purchases of high-GI foods.
3. **Scheduled meal prep time:** Dedicate specific times each week for meal preparation. This strategy will ease the cooking process, ensuring you always have healthy, diet-appropriate meals ready.
4. **Prepare ingredients in advance:** To simplify meal prep, wash, chop, and store fruits and vegetables ahead of time. Consider pre-cooking whole grains like brown rice or quinoa for easy use throughout the week.

SIMPLIFYING MEAL PREP WITH BATCH COOKING

Batch cooking involves preparing large quantities of food in advance, which aligns well with the Mediterranean and Reverse Type 2 Diabetes Diet principles. This approach can save time, lower the temptation for unhealthy convenience foods, and reduce stress.

UTILIZING KITCHEN TOOLS AND APPLIANCES

Investing in the right kitchen tools and appliances can streamline meal prep, making cooking more enjoyable and efficient.

By applying these cooking techniques and meal preparation strategies, you will create delicious, nutrient-dense, and low-GI meals that not only facilitate blood glucose control and weight loss but also promote diabetes reversal.

GUIDELINES FOR VEGETABLES AND VEGETABLE PRODUCTS

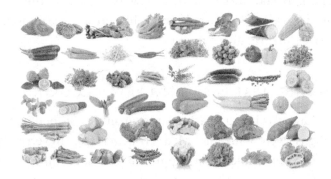

In the journey towards reversing Type 2 diabetes, every meal counts, and vegetables, a fundamental component of our diet, play an influential role. These nutrient-dense powerhouses offer us a path to improved health through their low glycemic index (GI) and high fiber content, placing them at the heart of the Reverse Type 2 Diabetes Diet.

This diet, a balanced fusion of the principles from the GI-GL approach, Mediterranean diet, and Dietary Guidelines for Americans 2020-2025, employs a strategic approach to food selection. It categorizes foods into five distinct groups with a significant emphasis on vegetables. These groups provide a roadmap for daily nutrition and ensure you are consuming a well-rounded mix of macro and micronutrients while keeping blood glucose levels stable.

A substantial component of this diet is the inclusion of low-glycemic load foods, particularly non-starchy and low-carbohydrate vegetables such as broccoli, asparagus, artichokes, and beets. The glycemic load considers both the quantity and quality of carbohydrates, and focusing on foods with a low glycemic load has been proven to better manage and even reverse Type 2 diabetes.

These vegetables, brimming with phytochemicals, vitamins, fiber, and minerals, are incredibly beneficial for individuals with diabetes. Green leafy vegetables, for instance, are packed with vitamin C and antioxidants - nutrients crucial for managing diabetes.

Studies have shown that individuals who adopt a diet high in low-glycemic load vegetables experience a variety of health benefits. These include weight loss, improved insulin sensitivity, and lower Hemoglobin A1c (HbA1c) levels, the latter being a vital marker of long-term blood glucose control.

In this chapter, you will gain valuable insights to confidently select, portion, and prepare these vegetables. By understanding their significant role in your diet and how to integrate them effectively into your meals, you can optimize their health benefits and move closer to your goal of reversing Type 2 diabetes.

UNDERSTANDING VEGETABLE PORTIONS:

Correct portion sizes form the foundation of meal planning. A single serving typically comprises 1 cup of raw vegetables or salad, ½ cup of cooked vegetables, and ¾ to 1 cup (6-8 oz) of unsweetened, home-made vegetable juice. For cooked beans, lentils, and peas, a serving size is ½ cup. Adjust these servings according to your appetite, caloric needs, and weight loss aspirations.

DAILY VEGETABLE INTAKE:

Strive for up to 10 daily servings across the five vegetable subgroups. This should encompass 1-2 servings of "Dark-Green Vegetables," 1-2 servings of "Red & Orange Vegetables," 1-2 servings of "Beans, Peas, Lentils," 2-3 servings of "Starchy Vegetables," and 2-3 servings of "Other Vegetables." A diverse intake ensures a comprehensive nutrient profile, leading to superior weight loss and blood glucose control outcomes.

EFFECTS OF COOKING ON THE GLYCEMIC INDEX OF VEGETABLES:

Cooking can alter the GI of vegetables by changing the structure and availability of carbohydrates, thus affecting the body's digestion and absorption rate. Here's how various cooking methods impact the GI:

- **Boiling and Steaming:** These methods maintain the low-GI value of vegetables by softening the fiber without significantly altering carbohydrate structure. However, avoid overcooking, which can raise the GI.
- **Roasting and Grilling:** These methods may slightly increase the GI due to caramelization, but the effect is typically negligible. Therefore, judiciously used roasted and grilled vegetables are an excellent component of a healthy, low-GI diet.
- **Baking:** Baking can slightly elevate the GI of starchy vegetables like potatoes. However, this increase doesn't categorize these foods as high-GI.
- **Microwaving:** Microwaving can marginally raise the GI of some vegetables, but not significantly, as it leads to minimal caramelization.
- **Frying:** This method can considerably increase the GI of vegetables as it can alter the food structure, allowing faster

carbohydrate absorption. Frying often incorporates fats or oils, increasing the overall calorie content.

Interestingly, the cooling of certain foods after boiling, like potatoes, pasta, and rice, triggers a process called retrogradation, which slows down digestion and lowers the GI.

INCREASING VEGETABLE INTAKE:

Here are some strategies to enhance your vegetable intake and improve blood sugar control:

- **Adding More Vegetables to Mixed Dishes:** Increasing your vegetable consumption doesn't have to be difficult or tedious. One easy way to include more vegetables in your diet is to add them to dishes you already enjoy. For example, if you're making a pasta dish, consider adding extra bell peppers, onions, zucchini, or spinach to the sauce.
- **Incorporating Vegetables into Breakfast:** Traditionally, breakfast in many cultures isn't very vegetable-heavy. However, there are many ways to change this. You could add spinach or other greens to your scrambled eggs or omelet, or even create a vegetable hash with sweet potatoes, bell peppers, and onions.
- **Blending Vegetables into Smoothies:** This can be a fantastic way to increase your vegetable intake, particularly if you or your family members aren't big fans of the taste of certain veggies. Leafy greens like kale, spinach, as well as vegetables like zucchini and cauliflower, can be easily added to smoothies without significantly changing the taste.
- **Preparing Vegetable-Based Sauces and Soups:** Soups and sauces offer an excellent way to consume a variety of vegetables in one meal. For example, a vegetable soup can be made with any veggies you have on hand, while a marinara sauce can include bell peppers, onions, and even carrots.

- **Opt for Fresh or Frozen Vegetables:** Fresh and frozen vegetables are typically free of added sugars and sodium, making them an optimal choice for a healthy diet. If fresh vegetables aren't available or affordable, frozen vegetables are a fantastic alternative. They are often frozen at peak ripeness, which helps preserve their nutrient content.
- **Pairing Vegetables with Protein and Healthy Fats:** This is a great tip. Including a protein source and healthy fats with your meals not only helps regulate blood sugar levels but can also make your meals more satisfying. This can promote weight loss by helping to prevent overeating.
- **Using the Food List:** Utilizing a detailed food list that provides the GI, sodium, potassium, and phosphorus values for various foods can indeed be a valuable tool. It can help you make informed decisions about which vegetables to include in your meals and how best to prepare them.
- **Vegetable Product Innovation:** Utilizing innovative vegetable-based products like spiralized vegetable noodles or cauliflower rice can help add variety to your meals while still maintaining blood sugar control and supporting weight loss efforts. Such products can often serve as direct replacements for more refined, higher-GI foods, helping you to transition more easily to a healthier eating pattern.

Remember, consistency is key. Start by integrating small changes into your diet, and over time, these will become new, healthier habits.

* * *

VEGETABLES AND VEGETABLE PRODUCTS:

Below are several vegetables and vegetable-based products that adhere to the guidelines of the Reverse Type 2 Diabetes Diet.

Leafy Greens and Cruciferous Vegetables:

• Arugula (Rocket) • Bok Choy • Brussels Sprouts • Cabbage • Cabbage Slaw • Chinese Broccoli (Gai Lan) • Collard Greens • Endive (Escarole) • Kale • Mustard Greens • Red Cabbage • Romaine Lettuce • Spinach • Swiss Chard • Turnip Greens • Water Spinach

Root Vegetables and Tubers:

• Beetroot • Butternut Squash • Carrots (Raw) • Jerusalem Artichoke • Jicama • Parsnips • Pumpkin • Radishes • Rutabaga (Swede) • Sweet Potatoes • Turnips

Nightshade and Fruit Vegetables:

• Aubergine (Eggplant) • Avocado • Capsicum (Bell Peppers) • Cucumbers • Okra • Tomatoes

Gourds and Squashes:

• Bottle Gourd • Butternut Squash • Pumpkin • Squash • Winter Melon • Zucchini (Courgette)

Bulb and Stem Vegetables:

• Asparagus • Celery • Fennel • Garlic • Leeks • Onions

Other Vegetables:

• • Mushrooms • Bamboo Shoots • Bean Sprouts • Green Beans • Snow Peas • Watercress • Daikon • Choy Sum • Kohlrabi • Bitter Gourd (Bitter Melon) • Radicchio • Artichokes

Canned Low GL Vegetables:

• Canned Artichokes • Canned Asparagus • Canned Beets • Canned Black Beans • Canned Carrots • Canned Green Beans • Canned

Green Peas • Canned Lentils • Canned Mushrooms • Canned Tomatoes

Fermented Vegetables:

• Fermented Beets • Fermented Cabbage (other than Kimchi and Sauerkraut) • Fermented Carrots • Fermented Cucumbers (pickles) • Fermented Garlic • Fermented Green Beans • Fermented Onions • Fermented Radishes • Kimchi • Sauerkraut

Low GL Vegetable Liquids:

• Butternut Squash Soup • Carrot Soup • Gazpacho Soup • Lentil Soup • Low-sodium Vegetable Broth • Miso Soup (with tofu and vegetables) • Pumpkin Soup • Spinach Soup • Tomato Juice (low sodium) • Zucchini Soup

Marinated Vegetables:

• Marinated Artichokes • Marinated Olives • Marinated Cucumbers • Marinated Beets • Marinated Eggplant • Marinated Onions • Marinated Mushrooms • Marinated Bell Peppers • Marinated Radishes • Marinated Zucchini

Vegetable Casseroles and Stews:

• Ratatouille • Baked Eggplant Parmesan • Lentil and Vegetable Casserole • Vegetable Pot Pie • Root Vegetable Stew • Vegetable Curry • Butternut Squash Casserole • Vegetable and Bean Chili • Vegetable and Barley Stew • • Sweet Potato and Black Bean Casserole

Pickled Vegetables:

• Pickled Cucumbers • Pickled Beets • Pickled Onions • Pickled

Carrots • Pickled Radishes • Pickled Green Beans • Pickled Okra • Pickled Asparagus • Pickled Garlic • Pickled Cauliflower

Vegetable Smoothies and Wraps:

• Spinach and Avocado Smoothie • Cucumber, Apple, and Kale Smoothie • Spinach, Cucumber, and Lemon Smoothie • Red Bell Pepper, Carrot, and Tomato Smoothie • Veggie Wrap with Avocado and Hummus • Veggie Wrap with Black Beans and Salsa • Veggie Wrap with Roasted Vegetables and Goat Cheese • Veggie Wrap with Lentils and Tahini Sauce• Veggie Wrap with Quinoa and Roasted Vegetables

Vegetable Condiments:

• Low-sodium Salsa • Guacamole • Pesto • Tomato Paste • Hummus • Baba Ganoush (eggplant dip) • Roasted Red Pepper Spread • Tzatziki

Remember to keep your preparation methods healthy too, such as grilling, roasting, and steaming, which preserve the vegetables' nutrient content and avoid adding unnecessary fats or sugars. Also, the overall meal's GI can be affected by what else is eaten with the vegetables. Furthermore, it is important to review the labels of canned or jarred vegetables to verify that they do not contain added sugars or excessive amounts of salt.

GUIDELINES FOR FRUITS AND FRUIT PRODUCTS

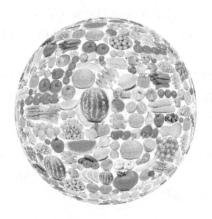

Fruits, much like vegetables, are crucial to Reverse Type 2 Diabetes Diet. They're generally rich in fiber and essential nutrients and typically have low to moderate GI values. Incorporating them into your meal plans can significantly contribute to optimal blood glucose control, overall health, and sustainable weight loss.

UNDERSTANDING FRUIT PORTIONS:

It's vital to understand the correct portion sizes for fruits. A serving of fruit typically equates to one medium piece, 1 cup of sliced fruits, or ½ cup (4 oz) of fruit juice.

Here are some general guidelines for what counts as a serving of fruit:

1. Fresh fruit: A serving size is generally about the size of a tennis ball or your fist. That's equivalent to a small apple, orange, or peach, or about 1/2 of a large banana.
2. Berries or cherries: A serving is 1 cup.
3. Grapes: A serving is about 15 grapes.
4. Dried fruit: Because drying fruit removes water and concentrates sugars, a serving size is smaller. For example, 2 tablespoons of raisins or dried cranberries is a serving.
5. Fruit Juice: Be careful with fruit juice, as it can have a lot of sugar and it doesn't contain the beneficial fiber found in whole fruit. A serving is 1/2 cup.
6. Canned or frozen fruit: For canned fruit, a serving size is 1/2 cup. Choose canned fruit that's packed in water or its own juice, not syrup. For frozen fruit, a serving is also typically 1/2 cup.

DAILY FRUIT INTAKE:

Strive to consume 2 to 4 servings of fruits daily. To maximize fiber intake and promote weight loss, at least 60% of your total fruit intake should come from whole fruits rather than 100% juice. When choosing juices, opt for those without added sugars or food additives.

UNDERSTANDING FRUIT RIPENESS:

The ripeness of a fruit can significantly influence its GL. As fruits ripen, their sugar content increases, thus raising their GI and GL. Therefore, less ripe fruits tend to have a lower GI. For instance, an unripe banana has a lower GI than a ripe one.

STRATEGIES TO INCREASE FRUIT INTAKE:

Here are some strategies to increase your fruit intake while improving blood sugar control:

- **Regular Consumption of Fruits:** Aim to include at least one serving of fruit in each of your meals. This doesn't necessarily mean eating a whole piece of fruit - it could be a handful of berries in your yogurt, slices of apple on your salad, or a side of melon with your dinner.
- **Adding Fruits to Breakfast:** Incorporating fruits into breakfast can make the meal more enjoyable while boosting its nutritional value. Add berries to your oatmeal, slices of banana to your cereal, or chopped fruit to your pancake batter. Avocado is a great addition to toast or eggs if you prefer savory breakfasts.
- **Choosing Whole Fruits as Snacks:** Whole fruits make excellent snacks as they're nutrient-rich, satisfying, and convenient. They provide fiber, which slows down the digestion of sugars and aids in keeping blood sugar levels stable. It's generally better to eat fruit whole rather than juiced to take full advantage of its fiber content.
- **Blending Fruits into Smoothies:** Similar to vegetables, you can effortlessly incorporate fruits into your diet by incorporating them into smoothies. This can be a fun and tasty way to consume a variety of fruits. To balance the sugar content, include a source of protein (e.g., Greek yogurt, protein powder) and healthy fats, like chia seeds or nut butter, in your smoothie.
- **Carrying Fruit for Later Consumption:** One of the biggest

challenges when trying to eat more fruits is convenience. You can have a healthy snack readily available when hunger strikes by simply carrying a piece of fruit with you, such as an apple or banana.

- Finding the Perfect Pairings with Your Favorite Foods: Fruits can also be paired with other foods to create satisfying meals or snacks. Pair apple slices with low-sodium cheese, spread nut butter on banana slices, or mix chopped fruit into cottage cheese or yogurt. Pairing fruit with a protein and/or fat source slows digestion and absorption of fruit sugars, which can aid maintain your blood sugar levels stable.

It's important to note that while fruits are nutritious, they do contain natural sugars and should be consumed as part of a balanced diet. Paying attention to portion sizes, especially for fruits that are higher in sugar or glycemic index, can help manage blood sugar levels effectively. By following these strategies and being mindful of your dietary needs and preferences, you can incorporate fruits into your Reverse Type 2 Diabetes Diet in a way that supports blood sugar control and overall health.

CHOOSING THE RIGHT FRUITS:

Prioritize fruits with a lower GI. Berries, cherries, peaches, apricots, apples, oranges, and pears are excellent choices for weight loss. Limit high-GI fruits like ripe bananas, pineapples, and watermelons.

CHOOSE WHOLE FRUITS OVER JUICES:

Whole fruits have more fiber and a lower GI than fruit juices. This makes them better for blood sugar control and weight management. If you choose to have juice, ensure it's 100% fruit juice, and limit your serving size to 4 ounces.

FRESH OR FROZEN FRUITS ARE BEST:

Fresh and frozen fruits with no added sugars are your optimal choice. If using canned or dried fruits, look for options with no added sugar, and adjust portion sizes, as these forms are more concentrated and could lead to excessive caloric intake.

PAIR FRUITS WITH PROTEIN OR HEALTHY FATS:

To slow glucose absorption and avoid blood sugar spikes, pair your fruits with a source of protein or healthy fats. This can also enhance satiety, supporting weight loss. For example, pair apple slices with a handful of nuts or serve berries with a portion of Greek yogurt.

USE THE EXTENSIVE FOOD LIST:

The food list provided in this book, which includes GI, GL, Net Carb values, is an invaluable tool for making informed decisions about which fruits and fruit products to include in your diet and in what quantities.

EXPERIMENT WITH FRUIT PRODUCTS:

Low-sugar fruit products, such as unsweetened applesauce or fruit spreads, can add variety to your diet, making it more enjoyable and sustainable. Always check the labels for added sugars to ensure they align with your weight loss goals.

* * *

FRUITS AND FRUIT PRODUCTS COMPLIANT WITH REVERSE TYPE 2 DIABETES DIET

Fresh and Frozen fruits:

• Apples • Oranges • Pears • Peaches • Plums • Cherries • Strawberries • Blueberries • Raspberries • Blackberries • Grapes • Kiwis • Nectarines • Papaya • Apricots • Grapefruit • Cantaloupe • Honeydew Melon • Watermelon • Guava • Avocado • Bananas (unripe) • Pomegranates • Boysenberries • Cranberries • Dragon fruit • Passion fruit • Goji Berries • Mulberries • Prunes • Pineapple • Lychee • Currants • Figs (fresh) • Lemons • Limes • Star Fruit • Elderberries • Gooseberries • Persimmons • Tangerines • Loganberries • Asian Pears • Acerola cherries

Dried Fruit

• Dried Apricots • Dried Apples • Dried Cherries • Dried Blueberries • Dried Prunes • Dried Dates (Each serving should not exceed 15 grams of carbohydrates.) • Dried Figs • Dried Pears • Dried Peaches • Dried Plums • Dried Cranberries • Dried Goji Berries • Dried Raisins • Dried Currants • Dried Strawberries • Dried Mulberries • Dried Nectarines • Dried Kiwi • Dried Mango (Each serving should not exceed 15 grams of carbohydrates.) • Dried Papaya • Dried Pineapple (Each serving should not exceed 15 grams of carbohydrates.) • Dried Bananas (Each serving should not exceed 15 grams of carbohydrates.) • Dried Coconut (Each serving should not exceed 15 grams of carbohydrates.) • Dried Guava • Dried Lychee • Dried Tangerines • Dried Passionfruit • Dried Pomegranate seeds • Dried Gooseberries • Dried Elderberries

Unsweetened frozen fruit mixes

• Mixed Berry Blend • Tropical Fruit Mix • Orchard Medley • Three-Berry Blend • Berry Cherry Mix • Citrus Blend • Berry Spinach Mix • Avocado Mango Mix • Cherry Almond Blend • Pomegranate Blueberry Mix • Pomegranate Blueberry Mix • Peach Raspberry Medley • Green Apple Berry Mix

Unsweetened fruit-based popsicles

• Berry Blast Popsicles • Tropical Sunshine Popsicles• Peachy Keen Popsicles • Melon Medley Popsicles • Kiwi Lime Popsicles • Cherry Vanilla Popsicles • Citrus Splash Popsicles • Apple Cinnamon Popsicles • Strawberry Basil Popsicles • Blueberry Lemonade Popsicles • Raspberry Mint Popsicles • Pomegranate Green Tea Popsicles • Apricot Almond Popsicles • Watermelon Lime Popsicles • Coconut Pineapple Popsicles • Cantaloupe Honey Popsicles • Pear Vanilla Popsicles

Fruit-based salsas

• Peach Salsa • Watermelon Salsa • Strawberry Salsa • Kiwi Salsa • Apple Salsa • Grape Salsa • Papaya Salsa • Pomegranate Salsa • Blueberry Salsa • Raspberry Salsa • Blackberry Salsa • Cranberry Salsa • Apricot Salsa • Guava Salsa • Plum Salsa • Nectarine Salsa • Lemon Salsa • Grapefruit Salsa

Fruit Products

• Apple sauce (unsweetened) • Fruit leather (no added sugar) • Fruit salads (without syrup) (Low GI, Low GL) • Homemade low-GL fruit smoothies • Fruit infused water • Low-sugar fruit jam • Fruit puree (no added sugar) • Fruit spread (unsweetened) • Unsweetened canned fruit in juice (not syrup) • Dehydrated fruit (no added sugar) • Fruit juice with pulp (Each serving should not exceed 15 grams of carbohydrates.)

Fruits used in Recipes

• Baked apples • Grilled peaches • Guacamole • Lemon zest Orange zest • Poached pears • Roasted low-GL fruit • Smoothie bowls with low GI fruits • Stewed apples without sugar • Strawberry puree (no added sugar) • Unsweetened apple butter (Low GI, Low GL)

Always remember, the portion size and what you eat with these fruits can affect their GI and GL. Pairing these fruits with proteins and fats can slow the absorption of sugars and reduce their GI.

GUIDELINES FOR GRAINS

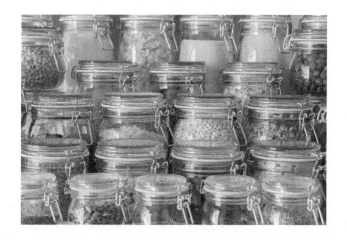

Grains are a significant food group with both benefits and risks for individuals seeking to reverse diabetes. Selection and consumption of grains require thoughtful consideration of factors like the Glycemic Index (GI), Glycemic Load (GL), the principles of the Mediterranean diet, and the Dietary Guidelines for Americans 2020-2025.

The Mediterranean diet values grains, particularly whole grains, for their rich dietary fiber, vitamins, minerals, and phytonutrients content. They contribute to balanced nutrition and overall health promotion. However, when it comes to diabetes reversal, not all grains provide equal benefits.

Refined grains, which have their bran and germ removed through a milling process, lose substantial nutritional value. Foods like white rice, white bread, and many processed cereals fall into this category. These products, with high GI and GL values, lead to rapid blood glucose spikes, posing challenges for diabetes management and reversal.

Even certain whole grains like brown rice or whole wheat bread, although nutritionally superior to refined grains, may have medium to high GI values. If not appropriately portioned or balanced with other foods, they could still cause blood sugar surges.

Thus, the importance of integrating Mediterranean diet principles with the GI-GL framework is highlighted for effective diabetes management. Reverse Type 2 Diabetes Diet cohesively combines these principles, addressing potential pitfalls and providing a comprehensive strategy for managing and possibly reversing diabetes.

Understanding the carbohydrate content of grains is crucial for diabetes meal planning. Typically, 15 grams of carbohydrates is considered one carb serving. However, it's essential to understand this may not align with common serving perceptions. For example, one cup of cooked rice, often perceived as a single serving, contains approximately 45 grams of carbohydrates, equivalent to three carb servings.

Given a target Glycemic Load (GL) of 50, corresponding to 50 grams of pure glucose, precise portion control of grains becomes vital.

This chapter aims to empower individuals to navigate the world of grains strategically, understanding the differences among grain types, their GI and GL values, and how they fit into a balanced diet aimed at reversing Type 2 diabetes. Equipped with this knowledge, individuals can enjoy the benefits of grains while effectively managing potential concerns, confidently progressing on the path to reversing Type 2 diabetes.

Choosing the Right Breakfast Cereals: When choosing breakfast cereals, opt for options made from whole grains that are low in sugar and high in fiber. Many breakfast cereals can be high in added sugars, which can increase their Glycemic Index (GI) and hinder weight loss efforts. Reading nutrition labels will assist in making informed choices.

Pair Grains with Protein and Healthy Fats: To balance the impact of grains on blood sugar levels, pair them with a source of protein and healthy fats. This combination can slow down glucose absorption and prevent blood sugar spikes. It also promotes satiety and supports weight loss. Consider having a slice of whole-grain bread with avocado and eggs for a nutritious and balanced breakfast.

Use the Food List: The extensive food list offered in parts IV and V of the book provides essential information such as the Glycemic Index (GI), Glycemic Load (GL) values, serving sizes, and net carb content. These valuable resources empower individuals to make informed decisions when including grains and breakfast cereals in their diet, helping them determine appropriate quantities for optimal weight management and overall well-being.

Understanding Portion Sizes: Knowledge of portion sizes is crucial. The typical serving sizes for cereals and grains include:

• ⅓ cup of breakfast cereal or muesli.

• ½ cup of cooked cereal or other cooked grain.

• ⅓ cup of cooked rice (excluding white rice).

• ½ cup of cold cereal.

All breakfast cereals in this list are low-glycemic-index and support a healthy weight.

Daily Grain Intake: Balance and variety are important for your daily grain intake. Aim for up to 3 servings per day, depending on your individual needs. Strategies to increase your intake of whole grains could involve:

• Replacing white bread with whole grain bread.

• Incorporating whole grains into salads or as a side dish.

• Choosing breakfast cereals made from whole grains.

The goal is to incorporate grains to support blood glucose control, overall health, and weight loss.

Grains and breakfast cereals can benefit a GI-focused diet when chosen and portioned correctly. Key steps include opting for whole grains, controlling portion sizes, and utilizing the provided food list. These guidelines can help you enjoy the benefits of grains and breakfast cereals while maintaining blood sugar control, supporting overall health, and promoting sustainable weight loss.

* * *

WHOLE GRAINS: THE SIMPLIFIED LIST

Here is the list of grains and cereals compliant with Reverse Type 2 Diabetes Diet

- Amaranth (all whole-grain products or used as ingredients)
- Barley (all whole-grain products or used as ingredients)
- Black rice (all whole-grain products or used as ingredients)
- Brown rice (all whole-grain products or used as ingredients)
- Buckwheat (all whole-grain products or used as ingredients)
- Bulgur (all whole-grain products or used as ingredients)
- Bulgur (cracked wheat) (all whole-grain products or used as ingredients)
- Cornmeal (whole grain) (all whole-grain products or used as ingredients)

- Dark rye (all whole-grain products or used as ingredients)
- Millet (all whole-grain products or used as ingredients)
- Multi-grain bread (all whole-grain products or used as ingredients)
- Multigrain couscous
- Oats (Avena sativa L.) (all whole-grain products or used as ingredients)
- Oats (steel-cut or rolled oats) (all whole-grain products or used as ingredients)
- Quinoa (all whole-grain products or used as ingredients)
- Sorghum (all whole-grain products or used as ingredients)
- Spelt (all whole-grain products or used as ingredients)
- Teff (all whole-grain products or used as ingredients)
- Whole grain bread (look for 100% whole wheat or other whole grains as the first ingredient)
- Whole grain corn (all whole-grain products or used as ingredients)
- Whole grain pasta (e.g., whole wheat, brown rice, quinoa)
- Whole grain rye (all whole-grain products or used as ingredients)
- Whole wheat (all whole-grain products or used as ingredients)
- Whole wheat couscous
- Whole-grain cereals (all whole-grain products or used as ingredients)
- Whole-wheat bread (all whole-grain products or used as ingredients)
- Whole-wheat chapati (all whole-grain products or used as ingredients)
- Wild rice (all whole-grain products or used as ingredients)

GUIDELINES FOR DAIRY AND PLANT-BASED ALTERNATIVES

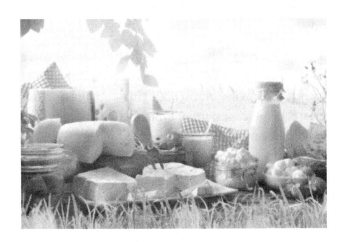

When it comes to meal planning, dairy products and plant-based alternatives play a significant role. This diverse food group includes traditional milk, cheese, and yogurt, as well as soy, almond, and other plant-based options. Incorporating dairy and plant-based alternatives into the diet has important implications for weight management, blood glucose control, and overall health. These choices align with principles such as the Glycemic Index (GI), Glycemic Load (GL), the

Mediterranean diet (MedDiet), and the Dietary Guidelines for Americans 2020-2025.

Research has shed light on the potential benefits of dairy products, particularly low-fat dairy and yogurt, in managing and potentially reversing type 2 diabetes. Studies published in esteemed journals such as the American Journal of Clinical Nutrition, Journal of Nutrition, European Journal of Epidemiology, and Diabetes Care have indicated a connection between higher consumption of low-fat dairy and improved insulin sensitivity, lower risk of type 2 diabetes, and better cardiometabolic profiles.

However, it's important to differentiate between different types of dairy products. Not all dairy plays a beneficial role in preventing type 2 diabetes. Specifically, low-fat dairy foods, especially yogurt, seem to offer the most advantages, while other dairy foods show no clear association.

Milk and other dairy products generally have a low glycemic load (GL) due to the moderate GI effect of lactose and the ability of milk protein to delay stomach emptying. This combination results in a slower release of glucose into the bloodstream, leading to a lesser impact on blood sugar levels compared to higher GI foods. Incorporating appropriate servings of dairy into the diet can contribute to better glycemic control, supporting diabetes management and reversal.

The role of dairy consumption in weight management is also significant. Weight loss is an essential aspect of the Reverse Type 2 Diabetes Diet, and when consumed in moderation and combined with regular physical activity, low-fat dairy products can support this goal.

Additionally, dairy products align with the principles of the Mediterranean diet, a globally recognized dietary pattern with well-established health benefits supported by scientific literature. The diet emphasizes the consumption of low-fat dairy products, which provide essential nutrients like calcium and protein, contributing to overall health and well-being.

However, what about plant-based alternatives? In addition to dairy products, plant-based alternatives play a crucial role in the Reverse Type 2 Diabetes Diet. These alternatives offer choices for individuals who prefer to limit or avoid dairy, have lactose intolerance, or follow a plant-based lifestyle. Plant-based alternatives include soy milk, almond milk, coconut milk, oat milk, and other non-dairy milk options.

In the context of managing and reversing type 2 diabetes, plant-based alternatives have several benefits. They typically contain lower amounts of saturated fat and cholesterol compared to traditional dairy products, which can be advantageous for cardiovascular health. Fortified plant-based milk alternatives can provide similar essential nutrients, as dairy milk.

Moreover, plant-based alternatives align with the principles of the Mediterranean diet and the Dietary Guidelines for Americans, which emphasize the inclusion of diverse protein sources, including plant-based options. Incorporating plant-based milk alternatives, along with other plant-based proteins like legumes, nuts, and seeds, supports a well-rounded diet that promotes overall health and aids in diabetes management.

When selecting plant-based alternatives for Reverse Type 2 Diabetes Diet, it is important to choose minimally processed options without added sugars. Reading labels and opting for unsweetened or low-sugar varieties is recommended. Additionally, ensuring adequate intake of nutrients typically found in dairy products (e.g., calcium, vitamin D), can be achieved by choosing fortified plant-based alternatives or incorporating other dietary sources of these nutrients.

By incorporating plant-based alternatives into Reverse Type 2 Diabetes Diet, you can enjoy a wide range of choices that align with their dietary preferences and support your goals for diabetes management.

* * *

Consider the following suggestions for incorporating dairy and non-dairy alternatives into Reverse Type 2 Diabetes Diet:

OPT FOR LOW-FAT AND NON-DAIRY ALTERNATIVES:

Choose low-fat or non-fat dairy products and fortified soy alternatives. These options generally have a lower GI and can participate in weight loss and overall health. Opt for unsweetened versions whenever possible to avoid added sugars, which can interfere with both blood sugar control and weight management.

CONSIDER PORTION SIZES:

A typical serving size for dairy and fortified soy alternatives is 1 cup of milk, yogurt, or 1.5 ounces of cheese. Controlling portion sizes is crucial for managing blood glucose levels and controlling calorie intake to support weight loss.

PAIR DAIRY WITH OTHER FOODS:

Pairing dairy products with other foods can help slow the absorption of glucose, maintain steady blood sugar levels, and enhance satiety, which is beneficial for weight loss. For example, you could pair a cup of reduced-fat yogurt with a handful of nuts and seeds for a balanced snack.

USE THE FOOD LIST:

Make use of the comprehensive food list provided in this guide. It includes information on GI, GL, and net carb values, helping you make informed decisions about which dairy products and fortified soy alternatives to include in your diet and in what quantities, while supporting weight loss.

DAILY DAIRY INTAKE:

Aim for 2-3 servings of dairy or fortified alternatives per day. This quantity can be adjusted based on individual dietary needs, preferences, and weight loss goals.

EXPERIMENT WITH DAIRY AND PLANT-BASED ALTERNATIVES:

Many different types of dairy products and fortified alternatives are available. Experimenting with these can add variety to your diet and make your meals more enjoyable while still contributing to weight loss.

By including plant-based alternatives in the Reverse Type 2 Diabetes Diet, you can enjoy a diverse array of choices that align with your dietary preferences and contribute to your goals of managing and reversing diabetes.

* * *

DAIRY AND FORTIFIED ALTERNATIVES: THE SIMPLIFIED LIST

Here is a list of dairy and fortified alternatives that are generally compliant with Reverse Type 2 Diabetes Diet, considering also their low sodium content:

Dairy Products:

- Low-fat or non-fat milk (cow's milk)
- Low-fat or non-fat milk (goat's milk)

- Greek yogurt (unsweetened, low-fat or non-fat)
- Skim milk powder
- Low-fat or non-fat cottage cheese
- Low-fat or non-fat plain yogurt
- Low-fat or non-fat kefir
- Low-fat or non-fat sour cream
- Low-fat or non-fat ricotta cheese
- Low-fat or non-fat cream cheese

Fortified Soy Alternatives:

- Unsweetened soy milk
- Unsweetened almond milk
- Unsweetened cashew milk
- Unsweetened oat milk
- Unsweetened rice milk
- Unsweetened coconut milk
- Unsweetened hemp milk
- Unsweetened pea protein milk

GUIDELINES FOR PROTEIN FOODS

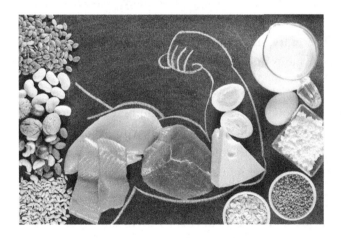

Transitioning to proteins is a crucial aspect of the Reverse Type 2 Diabetes Diet, as they are essential nutrients that support various biological functions in the body. Both animal-based and plant-based proteins play important roles in maintaining steady blood glucose levels, aiding in weight loss, and promoting overall health. These principles align with the Glycemic Index (GI) - Glycemic Load (GL) framework, the Mediterranean Diet (MedDiet), and the Dietary Guidelines for Americans 2020-2025.

It is important to understand the different subcategories within the protein food group, their unique benefits, and potential risks. Animal proteins, such as chicken, beef, pork, fish, eggs, and dairy, are primary sources of protein. Plant proteins include legumes, nuts, seeds, and whole grains. Both animal and plant proteins have a place in the Reverse Type 2 Diabetes Diet, but finding the right balance is key.

Numerous studies have shown that incorporating a variety of plant proteins alongside lean animal proteins can lead to greater reductions in serum cholesterol. This highlights the importance of including a diverse range of proteins, with a leaning towards plant-based sources, in line with the principles of the MedDiet.

It's essential to approach a high-protein diet with caution. While it may potentially benefit by improving HbA1c and liver fat content, high protein intake can strain the kidneys, especially in individuals with pre-existing Chronic Kidney Disease (CKD), even in its early stages. Therefore, moderation and balance are essential when incorporating proteins into a diet aimed at reversing type 2 diabetes.

It's also crucial to acknowledge the potential risks associated with insufficient protein intake. Not consuming enough protein can result in adverse effects such as muscle loss, compromised immune function, and various health complications. These consequences can negatively impact diabetes management and overall health.

The goal is to provide comprehensive guidance on how to optimally include proteins in the diet. This involves understanding the correct balance of animal and plant proteins, appropriate portion sizes, the importance of choosing lean and low-fat options, and incorporating proteins in a way that manages blood glucose levels, supports weight loss, and enhances overall health. With this knowledge, informed choices can be made to support the journey towards reversing type 2 diabetes.

* * *

Opt for Lean Proteins: Select lean protein sources like chicken breast, turkey, fish, eggs, and plant-based proteins like lentils, chickpeas, and tofu. Typically, these choices offer a low glycemic index (GI) and are crucial for promoting weight loss and maintaining good health. Be mindful of cooking methods; opt for grilling, broiling, or steaming rather than frying to avoid unnecessary fats and calories.

Consider Portion Sizes: A typical serving size for protein-rich foods is 3 ounces of cooked meat, poultry, or fish, 1 egg, 1/2 cup (125 g) of cooked beans, or 2 tablespoons of peanut butter. Controlling portion sizes is essential for managing blood glucose levels and controlling calorie intake to support weight loss.

Pair Protein with Other Foods: Pairing protein-rich foods with other nutritious foods can help maintain steady blood sugar levels and enhance satiety, which is beneficial for weight loss. For example, you could pair a grilled chicken breast with a serving of quinoa and colorful vegetables for a balanced meal.

Use the Food List: The comprehensive food list provided in this book, which includes GI, sodium, potassium, and phosphorus values, is an invaluable tool for making informed decisions about which protein-rich foods to include in your diet and in what quantities to support weight loss.

Daily Protein Intake: Aim for 2-3 servings of protein-rich foods per day. This quantity can be adjusted based on individual dietary needs, preferences, and weight loss goals.

Experiment with Protein Sources: Many different types of protein-rich foods are available, both animal-based and plant-based. Experimenting with these can add variety to your diet and make your meals more enjoyable while still contributing to weight loss.

These guidelines can help you enjoy the benefits of protein-rich foods while maintaining blood sugar control, supporting overall health, and promoting weight loss.

* * *

MEATS, POULTRY, EGGS: THE SIMPLIFIED LIST

Meats (lean or low-fats) include:

- beef, goat, lamb, and pork (fat red meats must be limited due to their pro-inflammatory effects). You have to choose lean meats preferably grass-fed beef, lamb, or bison
- game meat (e.g., bison, moose, elk, deer)

Poultry (lean or low-fats) includes

- chicken
- turkey
- cornish hens
- duck
- game birds (e.g., ostrich, pheasant, and quail)
- goose.

Eggs include

- chicken eggs
- turkey eggs
- duck eggs and other birds' eggs

* * *

SEAFOOD: THE SIMPLIFIED LIST

Seafood include

- salmon, sardine, anchovy, black sea bass, catfish, clams, cod, crab, crawfish, flounder, haddock, hake, herring, lobster, mullet, oyster, perch, pollock, scallop, shrimp, sole, squid, tilapia, freshwater trout, tuna

* * *

NUTS, SEEDS, SOY PRODUCTS: THE SIMPLIFIED LIST

Nuts (and nut butter) include

- almonds, pecans, Brazil nuts, pistachios, hazelnuts, macadamias, pine nuts, walnuts, cashew nuts

Seeds (and seed butter) include:

- pumpkin seeds, psyllium seeds, chia seeds, flax seeds, sunflower seeds, sesame seeds, poppy seeds

PART III
YOUR 30-DAY JOURNEY: A MEAL PLAN FOR SUCCESS

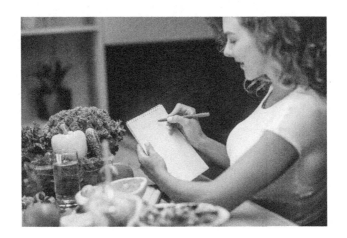

YOUR 30-DAY MEAL PLAN: AN OVERVIEW

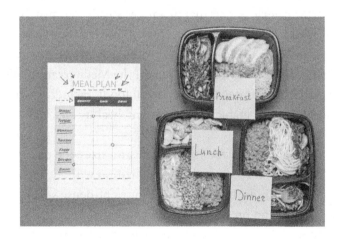

In your quest to reverse Type 2 Diabetes, having a clear action plan and dedication are key. To support you in this journey, we have developed a comprehensive 30-day meal plan that combines the principles of the Mediterranean diet, weight loss, caloric deficit, and Reverse Type 2 Diabetes Diet.

Our meal plan focuses on nutrient-dense, low-glycemic-index (GI), and low-glycemic-load (GL) foods to help manage and reverse diabetes by promoting gradual weight loss and improving blood glucose levels. The plan recognizes the significance of sustainable weight loss as the initial step towards diabetes reversal, and therefore creates a moderate caloric deficit that allows for healthy weight loss without deprivation. This approach directly impacts the pancreatic and liver fat cycles, crucial factors in Type 2 Diabetes.

Here's what you can expect from our 30-day meal plan:

- **Balanced Macronutrients:** The plan ensures an ideal balance of carbs, proteins, and fats, with a particular emphasis on complex carbs, lean proteins, and heart-healthy fats. This balance helps maintain consistent energy levels and optimize blood sugar control.
- **Caloric Deficit:** The plan is carefully designed to establish a moderate caloric deficit that promotes steady and sustainable weight loss. It's important to note that overly aggressive caloric deficits can have counterproductive effects.
- **Variety:** Embracing the principles of the Mediterranean diet, our plan incorporates a wide array of foods, including whole grains, fruits, vegetables, lean proteins, healthy fats, and legumes.
- **Portion Control:** By focusing on portion sizes, the plan ensures that you receive adequate nutrition without exceeding your caloric limits. It also includes nutrient-dense snacks to curb hunger and prevent overeating.
- **Seventeen Principles:** Our meal plan integrates the 17 principles of the Reverse Type 2 Diabetes Diet, providing a comprehensive approach to meal planning, preparation, and consumption. These principles will guide you in making healthy food choices, understanding portion sizes, and prioritizing low-GI and GL foods.
- **Nutrient-Dense Foods:** Prioritizing nutritional density, our plan includes an abundance of raw fruits, raw vegetables, and

whole grains. These foods are not only low-GL, but they also contribute to fiber intake and overall nutrient balance.

While our 30-day meal plan is meticulously crafted, we encourage you to adapt it to your individual caloric needs, dietary preferences, and any specific food allergies or intolerances. It serves as a solid foundation that you can customize to meet your unique requirements.

Remember, the journey towards Type 2 Diabetes reversal is personal, and our meal plan aims to support you by providing a holistic, nutritious, and enjoyable roadmap to improved health and well-being.

UNDERSTANDING AND ADAPTING YOUR MEAL PLAN: A PROGRESSIVE APPROACH

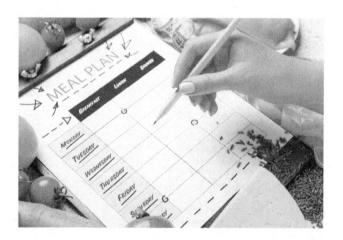

Understanding your body's unique nutritional needs is a crucial first step in adopting a new meal plan. This understanding begins with knowledge of the Basal Metabolic Rate (BMR)—the number of energy/calories your body requires to carry out basic functions while at rest, such as breathing and circulation. The BMR varies based on factors like age, sex, weight, and height.

To calculate your BMR accurately, you can utilize the BMR calculator provided by the National Institute of Health (NIH). This calculator employs the Mifflin-St. Jeor equation, which is a widely accepted formula for estimating BMR. The NIH BMR calculator is accessible through their website and is considered a reliable source. You will find it at the following link: https://www.niddk.nih.gov/bwp

Once you have determined your Basal Metabolic Rate (BMR), you can easily calculate your Total Daily Energy Expenditure (TDEE) by taking into account your activity level. The TDEE represents the total number of calories you need to maintain your current weight.

To calculate your TDEE, you can use the TDEE calculator provided by the National Institute of Health (NIH). This calculator takes into consideration factors such as age, sex, weight and height, and activity level to estimate your daily energy expenditure. The NIH TDEE calculator is available on their website at the following link: https://www.niddk.nih.gov/bwp

The 30-day meal plan is designed to be adaptable and can accommodate different calorie needs. The example provided for Day 1 includes a total of 2,000 calories. However, your caloric needs may be higher or lower based on your specific needs. For instance, if your TDEE is 2,500 calories but you aim for a caloric deficit, you might target a diet of 2,200 calories, promoting steady and sustainable weight loss. On the other hand, if your TDEE is only 1,800 calories, you would need to reduce portion sizes in the meal plan to meet that target.

To understand how to adapt the meal plan to your personal needs, let's walk through Day 1 of the plan:

Day 1:

- **Breakfast:** 1 cup of cooked steel-cut oats (150 cal), 1 cup of blueberries (85 cal), 1 tbsp of almond butter (98 cal) - Total: 333 cal
- **Lunch:** 150g of grilled chicken (300 cal), salad: 3 cups of mixed greens (45 cal), 1 cup of cherry tomatoes (27 cal), 1

cucumber (45 cal), 3 tbsp of vinaigrette (135 cal) - Total: 552 cal
- **Dinner:** 150g of baked salmon (360 cal), 1 cup of cooked quinoa (222 cal), 1.5 cups of steamed broccoli (80 cal) - Total: 662 cal
- **Snack 1:** 1 oz of mixed nuts (170 cal), 1 medium apple (95 cal) - Total: 265 cal
- **Snack 2:** 1 cup of carrot sticks (50 cal), 2 tbsp of hummus (50 cal) - Total: 100 cal

This day amounts to approximately 2,000 calories. If your daily caloric goal is 2,200 calories, you should add about 200 calories to this plan. This can be achieved by increasing portion sizes, adding an extra snack, or incorporating more calorie-dense foods like avocado or olive oil.

On the other hand, if your goal is 1,800 calories, you need to reduce the plan by around 200 calories. This adjustment could involve having a smaller portion of oats for breakfast, choosing a smaller piece of chicken for lunch, or reducing the number of nuts in the snack.

Remember, customization is key to a successful diet plan. Tailor the portions and food choices to your personal tastes and nutritional needs to make the plan enjoyable and sustainable. Embrace the journey of understanding your body's unique needs and how to nourish it effectively on your path to reversing Type 2 Diabetes.

WEEK 1: LAYING THE FOUNDATION

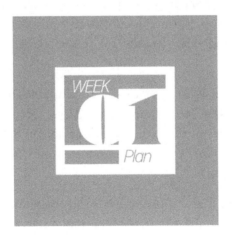

Welcome to the beginning of your transformative journey. The primary focus of this diet plan is to provide you with a valuable tool for effectively managing and potentially reversing type 2 diabetes while also promoting weight loss. It is important to understand that this plan integrates the principles of the Glycemic Index-Glycemic Load diet, the Mediterranean diet, and the Dietary Guidelines for Americans. These dietary frameworks are highly regarded for their effectiveness in controlling blood glucose levels, supporting heart health, managing weight, and promoting overall well-being.

During this first week, you will become acquainted with the strategic approach of combining foods with a low glycemic index and glycemic load. These dietary choices help stabilize your blood glucose levels, leading to a more balanced and healthier state for individuals with diabetes. Additionally, you will explore the rich and diverse palette of the Mediterranean diet, which emphasizes heart-healthy fats, lean proteins, and various fruits and vegetables.

It is important to note that you can customize this meal plan to suit your needs and preferences. While the plan provides a framework based on the principles of the Reverse Type 2 Diabetes Diet, it is not the only way to follow it. If you follow a specific dietary pattern or have particular dietary needs or preferences, such as being vegan or having celiac disease, you can substitute equivalent nutrient-dense, low-glycemic, and heart-healthy foods that better align with your requirements.

The ultimate goal is for you to feel comfortable in identifying and preparing foods that meet these criteria. As you become more familiar with the principles of the diet, you will be able to design a meal plan that works best for you, incorporating your favorite foods and recipes.

Please remember that this plan is just a starting point. It is designed to help you understand how to combine foods for optimal health and introduce you to a variety of dishes you may not have tried before. As you continue to learn and grow on your journey, you will discover that the best meal plan is the one you create for yourself within the framework of the Reverse Type 2 Diabetes Diet. Approach this journey with commitment and enthusiasm, and you will continue to make great progress toward your goals.

Here is the meal plan for the first week:

Day 1

- **Breakfast:** 1 cup of cooked steel-cut oats (170 cal), 1 cup of blueberries (85 cal), 1 tbsp of almond butter (98 cal), a drizzle of honey (21 cal) - Total: 374 cal
- **Lunch:** 150g of grilled chicken (165 cal), salad: 2 cups of mixed greens (15 cal), 1 cup of cherry tomatoes (27 cal), 1/2 cucumber (23 cal), 2 tbsp of olive oil vinaigrette (120 cal) - Total: 350 cal
- **Dinner:** 150g of baked salmon (280 cal), 1/2 cup of cooked quinoa (110 cal), 1 cup of steamed broccoli (55 cal) with a drizzle of extra virgin olive oil (60 cal) - Total: 505 cal
- **Snack 1:** 1 oz of mixed nuts (170 cal), 1 medium apple (95 cal)
- **Snack 2:** 1 cup of carrot sticks (50 cal), 2 tbsp of hummus (50 cal) - Total: 365 cal

Day 2

- **Breakfast:** 1 cup of Greek yogurt (150 cal), 1 cup of strawberries (50 cal), 1 tbsp of chia seeds (60 cal), a drizzle of honey (21 cal) - Total: 281 cal
- **Lunch:** 1 cup of lentil soup (220 cal), 1 slice of whole grain bread (80 cal), side of mixed greens with extra virgin olive oil dressing (50 cal) - Total: 350 cal
- **Dinner:** 150g of stir-fried tofu (180 cal), 1 cup of mixed vegetables (60 cal), cooked in 1 tbsp olive oil (120 cal) - Total: 360 cal
- **Snack 1:** 1 cup of Greek yogurt (150 cal), 10 almonds (70 cal)
- **Snack 2:** 1 cup of cucumber slices (15 cal), 2 tbsp of hummus (50 cal) - Total: 285 cal

Day 3

- **Breakfast:** 2 scrambled eggs (140 cal) with 1 cup of spinach (7 cal), 1 slice of whole grain toast (80 cal) drizzled with extra virgin olive oil (60 cal) - Total: 287 cal

- *Lunch:* 1 cup of quinoa salad with olive oil dressing (240 cal) with 1 cup of grilled vegetables (60 cal) - Total: 300 cal
- *Dinner:* 150g of grilled chicken breast (165 cal) with 1 tsp of olive oil (40 cal), 1 medium baked sweet potato (103 cal), 1 cup of green beans (31 cal) - Total: 339 cal
- *Snack 1:* 1 cup of cherry tomatoes (27 cal), 2 tbsp of hummus (50 cal)
- *Snack 2:* 1 medium apple (95 cal), 1 oz of cheddar cheese (110 cal) - Total: 282 cal

Day 4

- *Breakfast:* Smoothie with 2 cups of spinach (14 cal), 1 cup of blueberries (85 cal), 1 scoop of protein powder (100 cal), 1 tbsp of flaxseeds (55 cal) - Total: 254 cal
- *Lunch:* Whole grain sandwich with 3 oz of turkey (135 cal), 1 lettuce leaf (5 cal), 1 tomato slice (5 cal), 1/2 avocado (120 cal) - Total: 265 cal
- *Dinner:* 150g of baked cod with a drizzle of extra virgin olive oil (220 cal), 1 cup of steamed asparagus (40 cal), 1 cup of Greek salad (80 cal) - Total: 340 cal
- *Snack 1:* 2 medium peaches (120 cal), 10 almonds (70 cal)
- *Snack 2:* 1 cup of cottage cheese (220 cal), 1 tbsp of flaxseeds (55 cal) - Total: 465 cal

Day 5

- *Breakfast:* 2 poached eggs (140 cal), 1 cup of sautéed mushrooms in olive oil (100 cal), 1 slice of whole grain toast (80 cal) - Total: 320 cal
- *Lunch:* 1 cup of black bean soup (240 cal), 1 cup of mixed greens (15 cal), dressed with 1 tbsp of olive oil (120 cal) - Total: 375 cal
- *Dinner:* 150g of grilled shrimp (224 cal), 1/2 cup of cooked

brown rice (108 cal), 1 cup of Mediterranean salad (60 cal) - Total: 392 cal

- **Snack 1:** 1 cup of Greek yogurt (150 cal), 1 tbsp of honey (64 cal)
- **Snack 2:** 1 medium banana (105 cal), 1 tbsp of almond butter (98 cal) - Total: 417 cal

Day 6

- **Breakfast:** 1 cup of cooked quinoa (220 cal), 1 cup of almond milk (30 cal), 1 cup of mixed berries (70 cal) - Total: 320 cal
- **Lunch:** 1 whole grain wrap (210 cal) with 3 oz of tuna (99 cal), 1/2 cup of lettuce (3 cal), 2 slices of tomato (8 cal), 1 tbsp of olive oil (120 cal) - Total: 440 cal
- **Dinner:** 150g of roast turkey (240 cal), 1/2 cup of mashed sweet potato (103 cal), side of Greek salad (80 cal) - Total: 423 cal
- **Snack 1:** 1 cup of carrot sticks (50 cal), 2 tbsp of hummus (50 cal)
- **Snack 2:** 1 cup of grapes (104 cal), 1 oz of cheddar cheese (110 cal) - Total: 314 cal

Day 7

- **Breakfast:** 1 cup of Greek yogurt (150 cal), 1 cup of fresh peaches (60 cal), 1 tbsp of honey (64 cal) - Total: 274 cal
- **Lunch:** 150g of grilled chicken (165 cal), 2 cups of mixed salad (30 cal), 2 tbsp of vinaigrette (90 cal) - Total: 285 cal
- **Dinner:** 150g of baked salmon (280 cal), 1/2 cup of cooked quinoa (110 cal), 1 cup of steamed green beans with a drizzle of extra virgin olive oil (80 cal) - Total: 470 cal
- **Snack 1:** 1 medium apple (95 cal), 1 oz of mixed nuts (170 cal)
- **Snack 2:** 1 cup of cherry tomatoes (27 cal), 2 tbsp of cottage cheese (50 cal) - Total: 342 cal

This week's menu is thoughtfully crafted, incorporating lean proteins, heart-healthy fats, and a wide variety of fruits and vegetables. All the while, we've kept the calorie count in check to ensure that you are creating a caloric deficit for effective weight loss. Enjoy the flavors of the Mediterranean diet while working towards your goal of reversing type 2 diabetes.

WEEK 2: FORMING NEW HABITS

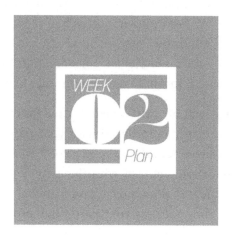

Greetings as you progress into the second week of this transformative endeavor. Thus far, you have initiated significant strides toward enhancing your health by adopting a lifestyle centered around nutrient-dense, low-glycemic, and heart-healthy foods. This week, we shall further explore this harmonious dietary approach, which serves as a vehicle driving you closer to the dual objectives of this plan: reversing type 2 diabetes and achieving sustainable weight loss.

As we advance through the week, the Mediterranean diet's influence will persist, enriching your meals with vibrant flavors and aligning seamlessly with our mission. Prioritizing whole grains, lean proteins, healthy fats, and an array of fruits and vegetables, your diet is being tailored for effective blood sugar control, weight management, and enhanced cardiovascular health.

It's important to note that the plan we present is intended as a robust foundation, a kickstarter, if you will, rather than a rigid prescription. The ultimate goal is for you to become well-versed in the principles and spirit of the Reverse Type 2 Diabetes Diet and the friendly foods, cooking methods, and portion sizes that it encompasses. With this knowledge, you will be empowered to adapt the plan to meet your individual dietary needs and preferences.

This is particularly relevant if you are following a vegan diet, have celiac disease, or any food intolerance. While the broad structure of the plan remains valid, the specific food choices may need to be adjusted to align with these dietary considerations. Remember, this plan is adaptable and is meant to guide you rather than constrain you.

The diet plan that will be most beneficial and sustainable for you is the one that is crafted in accordance with your personal preferences but within the framework of the Reverse Type 2 Diabetes Diet. As you progress and familiarize yourself with this new dietary lifestyle, you will become proficient in designing a meal plan that is tailor-made for you, one that not only satisfies your palate but also aligns with your health objectives.

Let's progress further on this journey, with the understanding that this diet plan is not a set formula but a dynamic and adaptable tool to aid your path towards better health.

Day 8

- **Breakfast:** 1 cup of oatmeal (150 cal), 1 medium banana (105 cal), 1 tbsp of honey (64 cal) - Total: 319 cal

- *Lunch:* Salad with 2 cups of mixed greens (15 cal), 1/2 cup of chickpeas (134 cal), 1/2 cup of cherry tomatoes (27 cal), 1/2 cup of cucumber (8 cal), 2 tbsp of extra virgin olive oil (240 cal) - Total: 424 cal
- *Dinner:* 150g of grilled chicken breast (165 cal), 1 cup of steamed vegetables (60 cal), 1/2 cup of cooked quinoa (110 cal) - Total: 335 cal
- *Snack 1:* 1 medium apple (95 cal), 1 oz of almonds (160 cal)
- *Snack 2:* 1 cup of Greek yogurt (150 cal), 1 tbsp of chia seeds (60 cal), 10 almonds (70 cal) - Total: 335 cal

Day 9

- *Breakfast:* 2 scrambled eggs (140 cal), 1 slice of whole grain toast (80 cal), 1/2 avocado (120 cal) - Total: 340 cal
- *Lunch:* 1 cup of lentil soup (220 cal), 1 slice of whole grain bread (80 cal), 1 cup of cucumber slices (16 cal), 2 tbsp of hummus (50 cal) - Total: 366 cal
- *Dinner:* 150g of baked cod (189 cal), 1 cup of steamed broccoli (55 cal), 1/2 cup of cooked quinoa (110 cal) - Total: 354 cal
- *Snack 1:* 1 medium orange (62 cal), 10 walnuts (183 cal)
- *Snack 2:* 1 cup of cherry tomatoes (27 cal), 2 tbsp of hummus (50 cal) - Total: 322 cal

Day 10

- *Breakfast:* Smoothie with 1 cup of almond milk (30 cal), 1 banana (105 cal), 1 scoop of protein powder (100 cal), 1 cup of spinach (7 cal), 1 tbsp of chia seeds (60 cal) - Total: 302 cal
- *Lunch:* Salad with 2 cups of spinach (14 cal), 1/2 cup of cherry tomatoes (27 cal), 1 boiled egg (70 cal), 1/2 cup of roasted sweet potato cubes (90 cal), 2 tbsp of extra virgin olive oil (240 cal) - Total: 441 cal
- *Dinner:* 150g of grilled shrimp (224 cal), 1 cup of steamed

green beans (44 cal), 1/2 cup of cooked brown rice (108 cal) - Total: 376 cal
- *Snack 1:* 1 cup of Greek yogurt (150 cal), 1 tbsp of honey (64 cal)
- *Snack 2:* 1 medium apple (95 cal), 1 oz of cheddar cheese (110 cal) - Total: 319 cal

Day 11

- *Breakfast:* 2 poached eggs (140 cal), 1 slice of whole grain toast (80 cal), 1/2 avocado (120 cal) - Total: 340 cal
- *Lunch:* 1 cup of vegetable soup (100 cal), 1 slice of whole grain bread (80 cal), 3 oz of turkey (135 cal), 1 cup of cucumber slices (16 cal), 2 tbsp of hummus (50 cal) - Total: 381 cal
- *Dinner:* 150g of grilled salmon (280 cal), 1 cup of steamed asparagus (40 cal), 1/2 cup of cooked quinoa (110 cal) - Total: 430 cal
- *Snack 1:* 1 medium orange (62 cal), 10 walnuts (183 cal)
- *Snack 2:* 1 cup of cherry tomatoes (27 cal), 2 tbsp of hummus (50 cal) - Total: 322 cal

Day 12

- *Breakfast:* 1 cup of oatmeal (150 cal), 1 medium banana (105 cal), 1 tbsp of chia seeds (60 cal) - Total: 315 cal
- *Lunch:* Salad with 2 cups of mixed greens (15 cal), 1/2 cup of black beans (120 cal), 1/2 cup of cherry tomatoes (27 cal), 1/2 cup of corn (89 cal), 2 tbsp of extra virgin olive oil (240 cal) - Total: 491 cal
- *Dinner:* 150g of roasted turkey (240 cal), 1 cup of steamed vegetables (60 cal), 1/2 cup of cooked quinoa (110 cal) - Total: 410 cal
- *Snack 1:* 1 medium apple (95 cal), 1 oz of almonds (160 cal)
- *Snack 2:* 1 cup of Greek yogurt (150 cal), 1 cup of mixed berries (70 cal), 10 almonds (70 cal) - Total: 380 cal

Day 13

- **Breakfast:** 1 cup of Greek yogurt (150 cal), 1 cup of fresh pineapple (82 cal), 1 tbsp of honey (64 cal) - Total: 296 cal
- **Lunch:** 1 cup of tomato soup (150 cal), 1 slice of whole grain bread (80 cal), 1/2 avocado (120 cal) - Total: 350 cal
- **Dinner:** 150g of grilled chicken (165 cal), 1 cup of steamed Brussels sprouts (56 cal), 1/2 cup of cooked quinoa (110 cal) - Total: 331 cal
- **Snack 1:** 1 medium orange (62 cal), 10 walnuts (183 cal)
- **Snack 2:** 1 cup of cherry tomatoes (27 cal), 2 tbsp of hummus (50 cal) - Total: 322 cal

Day 14

- **Breakfast:** Smoothie with 1 cup of almond milk (30 cal), 1 cup of spinach (7 cal), 1 banana (105 cal), 1 scoop of protein powder (100 cal), 1 tbsp of chia seeds (60 cal) - Total: 302 cal
- **Lunch:** Salad with 2 cups of spinach (14 cal), 1 boiled egg (70 cal), 1/2 cup of cherry tomatoes (27 cal), 1/2 cup of roasted sweet potato cubes (90 cal), 2 tbsp of extra virgin olive oil (240 cal) - Total: 441 cal
- **Dinner:** 150g of baked cod (189 cal), 1 cup of steamed broccoli (55 cal), 1/2 cup of cooked quinoa (110 cal) - Total: 354 cal
- **Snack 1:** 1 cup of Greek yogurt (150 cal), 1 tbsp of honey (64 cal)
- **Snack 2:** 1 medium apple (95 cal), 1 oz of cheddar cheese (110 cal) - Total: 319 cal

WEEK 3: TAILORING YOUR APPROACH

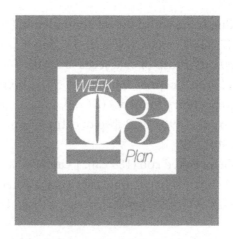

As you progress into the third week, it is essential to acknowledge the growth in your understanding and awareness of nutrition for managing and potentially reversing type 2 diabetes. By now, you should have a solid grasp on what foods to embrace, what to limit, and how to balance meals that improve insulin sensitivity. Moreover, you're becoming adept at creating a meal plan that supports weight loss and fosters a caloric deficit.

Creating a realistic caloric deficit is a key factor in this journey. A caloric deficit happens when you consume fewer calories than your body uses, leading to weight loss. This strategy, however, should be implemented carefully and realistically to ensure it's sustainable over the long term.

To help guide your weight loss journey, focus on reaching a healthy body mass index (BMI). If you're overweight, aim for a weight loss of at least 8 kg. For those who are obese, aim for a loss of 14 kg or more. However, remember that these targets are general guidelines, and individual weight loss goals may vary.

Remember that weight loss often takes time, and significant changes may not be immediately visible. The most meaningful weight loss is the one that you can maintain over the long term. Rapid weight loss might be tempting, but it's often harder to sustain and may not be healthy.

As you continue on this transformative journey, embrace the process of learning and adapting. Stay dedicated to the principles of the Reverse Type 2 Diabetes Diet, and you'll discover how to create a personalized nutrition strategy that aligns with your health goals, preferences, and lifestyle. This week, take the opportunity to explore, learn, and savor the flavors of healthy eating. With each passing day, you'll move closer to achieving your goals and enjoying the rewards of improved health.

Day 15

- *Breakfast:* 2 scrambled eggs (140 cal), 1 slice of whole grain toast (80 cal), 1/2 avocado (120 cal) - Total: 340 cal
- *Lunch:* 1 cup of lentil soup (220 cal), 1 slice of whole grain bread (80 cal) - Total: 300 cal
- *Dinner:* 150g of grilled shrimp (224 cal), 1 cup of steamed green beans (44 cal), 1/2 cup of cooked quinoa (110 cal) - Total: 378 cal
- *Snack 1:* 1 medium apple (95 cal), 1 oz of almonds (160 cal)

- **Snack 2:** 1 cup of Greek yogurt (150 cal), 1 tbsp of chia seeds (60 cal) - Total: 305 cal

Day 16

- **Breakfast:** Smoothie with 1 cup of almond milk (30 cal), 1 small banana (105 cal), 1 scoop of protein powder (100 cal), 1 cup of spinach (7 cal) - Total: 242 cal
- **Lunch:** Salad with 2 cups of mixed greens (15 cal), 1/2 cup of cherry tomatoes (27 cal), 1 boiled egg (70 cal), 1/2 cup of roasted sweet potato cubes (90 cal), 2 tbsp of vinaigrette (90 cal) - Total: 292 cal
- **Dinner:** 150g of grilled salmon (280 cal), 1 cup of steamed asparagus (40 cal), 1/2 cup of cooked brown rice (108 cal) - Total: 428 cal
- **Snack 1:** 1 medium orange (62 cal), 1 oz of mixed nuts (170 cal)
- **Snack 2:** 1 cup of carrot sticks (50 cal), 2 tbsp of hummus (50 cal) - Total: 282 cal

Day 17

- **Breakfast:** 2 poached eggs (140 cal), 1 slice of whole grain toast (80 cal), 1/2 avocado (120 cal) - Total: 340 cal
- **Lunch:** 1 cup of vegetable soup (100 cal), 1 slice of whole grain bread (80 cal), 1 oz of turkey (50 cal) - Total: 230 cal
- **Dinner:** 150g of roasted turkey (240 cal), 1 cup of steamed vegetables (60 cal), 1/2 cup of cooked quinoa (110 cal) - Total: 410 cal
- **Snack 1:** 1 medium apple (95 cal), 1 oz of almonds (160 cal)
- **Snack 2:** 1 cup of Greek yogurt (150 cal), 1 cup of mixed berries (70 cal) - Total: 315 cal

Day 18

- **Breakfast:** 1 cup of oatmeal (150 cal), 1 medium banana (105 cal), 1 tbsp of chia seeds (60 cal) - Total: 315 cal
- **Lunch:** Salad with 2 cups of mixed greens (15 cal), 1/2 cup of black beans (120 cal), 1/2 cup of cherry tomatoes (27 cal), 1/2 cup of corn (89 cal), 2 tbsp of vinaigrette (90 cal) - Total: 341 cal
- **Dinner:** 150g of baked cod (189 cal), 1 cup of steamed broccoli (55 cal), 1/2 cup of cooked brown rice (108 cal) - Total: 352 cal
- **Snack 1:** 1 medium orange (62 cal), 1 oz of mixed nuts (170 cal)
- **Snack 2:** 1 cup of carrot sticks (50 cal), 2 tbsp of hummus (50 cal) - Total: 282 cal

Day 19

- **Breakfast:** 1 cup of Greek yogurt (150 cal), 1 cup of fresh pineapple (82 cal), 1 tbsp of honey (64 cal) - Total: 296 cal
- **Lunch:** 1 cup of tomato soup (150 cal), 1 slice of whole grain bread (80 cal) - Total: 230 cal
- **Dinner:** 150g of grilled chicken (165 cal), 1 cup of steamed Brussels sprouts (56 cal), 1/2 cup of cooked quinoa (110 cal) - Total: 331 cal
- **Snack 1:** 1 medium apple (95 cal), 1 oz of almonds (160 cal)
- **Snack 2:** 1 cup of Greek yogurt (150 cal), 1 tbsp of chia seeds (60 cal) - Total: 305 cal

Day 20

- **Breakfast:** Smoothie with 1 cup of almond milk (30 cal), 1 cup of spinach (7 cal), 1 banana (105 cal), 1 scoop of protein powder (100 cal) - Total: 242 cal
- **Lunch:** Salad with 2 cups of spinach (14 cal), 1 boiled egg (70 cal), 1/2 cup of cherry tomatoes (27 cal), 1/2 cup of roasted sweet potato cubes (90 cal), 2 tbsp of vinaigrette (90 cal) - Total: 291 cal

- *Dinner:* 150g of grilled shrimp (224 cal), 1 cup of steamed green beans (44 cal), 1/2 cup of cooked quinoa (110 cal) - Total: 378 cal
- *Snack 1:* 1 medium orange (62 cal), 1 oz of mixed nuts (170 cal)
- *Snack 2:* 1 cup of carrot sticks (50 cal), 2 tbsp of hummus (50 cal) - Total: 282 cal

Day 21

- *Breakfast:* 2 scrambled eggs (140 cal), 1 slice of whole grain toast (80 cal), 1/2 avocado (120 cal) - Total: 340 cal
- *Lunch:* 1 cup of lentil soup (220 cal), 1 slice of whole grain bread (80 cal) - Total: 300 cal
- *Dinner:* 150g of grilled salmon (280 cal), 1 cup of steamed asparagus (40 cal), 1/2 cup of cooked brown rice (108 cal) - Total: 428 cal
- *Snack 1:* 1 medium apple (95 cal), 1 oz of almonds (160 cal)
- *Snack 2:* 1 cup of Greek yogurt (150 cal), 1 tbsp of chia seeds (60 cal) - Total: 305 cal

WEEK 4: CONSISTENCY IS KEY

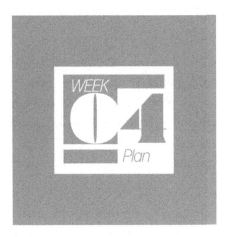

As you embark on the fourth week of this health transformation journey, it's time to focus on personalizing your diet even more. This personalization is an essential aspect of long-term success. You've spent the past weeks learning about the principles of a diet that can aid in reversing type 2 diabetes and promote weight loss. Now, you're beginning to see health improvements, experience weight loss, and gain a heightened awareness of how your body responds to different foods.

Protein intake is a crucial aspect of your diet. It's important to maintain a healthy level of protein to prevent muscle loss, a common issue for individuals with diabetes. Quality protein sources include lean meats, fish, eggs, dairy, and plant-based alternatives such as lentils, chickpeas, and tofu. Adjust your protein intake according to your personal needs, preferences, and the advice of your healthcare provider.

By this point, you might start to notice some changes in your health markers. Blood tests could show improvements in your Hemoglobin A1c (HbA1c), which gives an indication of your average blood glucose levels over the past two to three months. You may also notice improvements in your lipid profile, including levels of LDL ("bad") cholesterol, HDL ("good") cholesterol, and triglycerides. These improvements are signs that your body is responding well to the dietary changes, and they're also markers of reduced risk for cardio-vascular diseases.

Now that you've laid down a solid foundation and begun experiencing some of the benefits of your new dietary habits, it's time to personalize your meal plan. This is not a one-size-fits-all journey. Each individual's path to health will look different. Some people might prefer a diet rich in certain types of food, while others may have dietary restrictions or ethical considerations that influence their choices.

Personalization might mean adjusting portion sizes, experimenting with new foods or recipes, or tweaking meal timing to better fit your lifestyle. Always keep in mind that the overarching objective is to construct a sustainable plan that suits you in the long run. This entails creating a plan that brings you enjoyment, seamlessly integrates into your daily routine, and consistently propels you towards achieving your health goals.

Day 22

- *Breakfast:* Smoothie with 1 cup of almond milk (30 cal), 1 cup of mixed berries (70 cal), 1 scoop of protein powder (100 cal), 1 cup of spinach (7 cal) - Total: 207 cal

- **Lunch:** 1 cup of chicken soup (150 cal), 1 slice of whole grain bread (80 cal) - Total: 230 cal
- **Dinner:** 150g of grilled tofu (144 cal), 1 cup of stir-fried mixed vegetables (150 cal), 1/2 cup of cooked brown rice (108 cal) - Total: 402 cal
- **Snack 1:** 1 medium pear (102 cal), 1 oz of almonds (160 cal)
- **Snack 2:** 1 cup of Greek yogurt (150 cal), 1 tbsp of chia seeds (60 cal) - Total: 310 cal

Day 23

- **Breakfast:** 2 boiled eggs (140 cal), 1 slice of whole grain toast (80 cal), 1/2 avocado (120 cal) - Total: 340 cal
- **Lunch:** Salad with 2 cups of mixed greens (15 cal), 1/2 cup of chickpeas (135 cal), 1/2 cup of cherry tomatoes (27 cal), 1/2 cup of cucumber (8 cal), 2 tbsp of vinaigrette (90 cal) - Total: 275 cal
- **Dinner:** 150g of baked salmon (280 cal), 1 cup of steamed green beans (44 cal), 1/2 cup of cooked quinoa (110 cal) - Total: 434 cal
- **Snack 1:** 1 medium apple (95 cal), 1 oz of mixed nuts (170 cal)
- **Snack 2:** 1 cup of carrot sticks (50 cal), 2 tbsp of hummus (50 cal) - Total: 285 cal

Day 24

- **Breakfast:** 1 cup of oatmeal (150 cal), 1 cup of fresh strawberries (49 cal), 1 tbsp of honey (64 cal) - Total: 263 cal
- **Lunch:** 1 cup of vegetable soup (100 cal), 1 slice of whole grain bread (80 cal), 1 oz of turkey (50 cal) - Total: 230 cal
- **Dinner:** 150g of grilled chicken (165 cal), 1 cup of steamed Brussels sprouts (56 cal), 1/2 cup of cooked brown rice (108 cal) - Total: 329 cal

- **Snack 1:** 1 medium banana (105 cal), 1 oz of almonds (160 cal)
- **Snack 2:** 1 cup of Greek yogurt (150 cal), 1 cup of fresh blueberries (85 cal) - Total: 335 cal

Day 25

- **Breakfast:** Smoothie with 1 cup of almond milk (30 cal), 1 banana (105 cal), 1 scoop of protein powder (100 cal), 1 cup of kale (36 cal) - Total: 271 cal
- **Lunch:** Salad with 2 cups of spinach (14 cal), 1 boiled egg (70 cal), 1/2 cup of cherry tomatoes (27 cal), 1/2 cup of roasted sweet potato cubes (90 cal), 2 tbsp of vinaigrette (90 cal) - Total: 291 cal
- **Dinner:** 150g of grilled shrimp (224 cal), 1 cup of steamed broccoli (55 cal), 1/2 cup of cooked quinoa (110 cal) - Total: 389 cal
- **Snack 1:** 1 medium orange (62 cal), 1 oz of mixed nuts (170 cal)
- **Snack 2:** 1 cup of carrot sticks (50 cal), 2 tbsp of hummus (50 cal) - Total: 282 cal

Day 26

- **Breakfast:** 2 scrambled eggs (140 cal), 1 slice of whole grain toast (80 cal), 1/2 avocado (120 cal) - Total: 340 cal
- **Lunch:** 1 cup of lentil soup (220 cal), 1 slice of whole grain bread (80 cal) - Total: 300 cal
- **Dinner:** 150g of grilled salmon (280 cal), 1 cup of steamed asparagus (40 cal), 1/2 cup of cooked brown rice (108 cal) - Total: 428 cal
- **Snack 1:** 1 medium apple (95 cal), 1 oz of almonds (160 cal)
- **Snack 2:** 1 cup of Greek yogurt (150 cal), 1 tbsp of chia seeds (60 cal) - Total: 305 cal

Day 27

- **Breakfast:** 1 cup of Greek yogurt (150 cal), 1 cup of fresh pineapple (82 cal), 1 tbsp of honey (64 cal) - Total: 296 cal
- **Lunch:** 1 cup of tomato soup (150 cal), 1 slice of whole grain bread (80 cal) - Total: 230 cal
- **Dinner:** 150g of grilled chicken (165 cal), 1 cup of steamed Brussels sprouts (56 cal), 1/2 cup of cooked quinoa (110 cal) - Total: 331 cal
- **Snack 1:** 1 medium apple (95 cal), 1 oz of almonds (160 cal)
- **Snack 2:** 1 cup of Greek yogurt (150 cal), 1 tbsp of chia seeds (60 cal) - Total: 305 cal

Day 28

- **Breakfast:** Smoothie with 1 cup of almond milk (30 cal), 1 cup of spinach (7 cal), 1 banana (105 cal), 1 scoop of protein powder (100 cal) - Total: 242 cal
- **Lunch:** Salad with 2 cups of spinach (14 cal), 1 boiled egg (70 cal), 1/2 cup of cherry tomatoes (27 cal), 1/2 cup of roasted sweet potato cubes (90 cal), 2 tbsp of vinaigrette (90 cal) - Total: 291 cal
- **Dinner:** 150g of grilled shrimp (224 cal), 1 cup of steamed green beans (44 cal), 1/2 cup of cooked quinoa (110 cal) - Total: 378 cal
- **Snack 1:** 1 medium orange (62 cal), 1 oz of mixed nuts (170 cal)
- **Snack 2:** 1 cup of carrot sticks (50 cal), 2 tbsp of hummus (50 cal) - Total: 282 cal

Day 29

- **Breakfast:** 2 poached eggs (140 cal), 1 slice of whole grain toast (80 cal), 1/2 avocado (120 cal) - Total: 340 cal
- **Lunch:** 1 cup of vegetable soup (100 cal), 1 slice of whole grain bread (80 cal), 3 oz of turkey (135 cal), 1 cup of cucumber slices (16 cal), 2 tbsp of hummus (50 cal) - Total: 381 cal

- **Dinner:** 150g of grilled salmon (280 cal), 1 cup of steamed asparagus (40 cal), 1/2 cup of cooked quinoa (110 cal) - Total: 430 cal
- **Snack 1:** 1 medium orange (62 cal), 10 walnuts (183 cal)
- **Snack 2:** 1 cup of cherry tomatoes (27 cal), 2 tbsp of hummus (50 cal) - Total: 322 cal

Day 30

- **Breakfast:** 1 cup of Greek yogurt (150 cal), 1 cup of fresh peaches (60 cal), 1 tbsp of honey (64 cal) - Total: 274 cal
- **Lunch:** 150g of grilled chicken (165 cal), 2 cups of mixed salad (30 cal), 2 tbsp of vinaigrette (90 cal) - Total: 285 cal
- **Dinner:** 150g of baked salmon (280 cal), 1/2 cup of cooked quinoa (110 cal), 1 cup of steamed green beans with a drizzle of extra virgin olive oil (80 cal) - Total: 470 cal
- **Snack 1:** 1 medium apple (95 cal), 1 oz of mixed nuts (170 cal)
- **Snack 2:** 1 cup of cherry tomatoes (27 cal), 2 tbsp of cottage cheese (50 cal) - Total: 342 cal

PART IV
YOUR GO-TO GUIDE: BEST FOODS FOR THE TYPE 2 DIABETES REVERSAL DIET

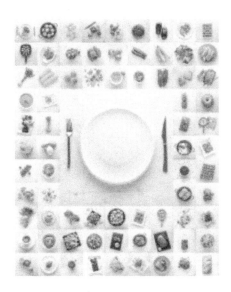

AMERICAN RESTAURANT FOODS

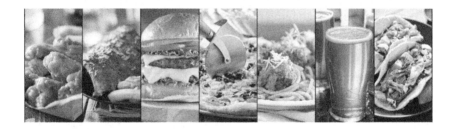

The wide range of American restaurant foods can play a part in the diets of many individuals, including those pursuing Reverse Type 2 Diabetes Diet. The critical evaluation of their inclusion involves assessing their glycemic load (GL), nutritional content, and fit within Reverse Type 2 Diabetes Diet. Understanding American restaurant foods' benefits and potential drawbacks can empower individuals to make knowledgeable dietary choices that support diabetes management and overall health.

Benefits of American Restaurant Foods:

- **Diverse Options:** American restaurant foods offer a wide range of choices, from salads and grilled proteins to whole grain options and vegetable-based dishes.

- **Potential for Balanced Meals:** Many restaurants offer options that can be tailored to fit within a Reverse Type 2 Diabetes Diet, including lean proteins, whole grains, and vegetables.

Potential Drawbacks of American Restaurant Foods:

- **High in Calories and Carbs:** Many American restaurant foods are high in calories and carbohydrates. These foods can quickly exceed the recommended daily intake for individuals with type 2 diabetes, leading to blood sugar spikes.
- **Large Portions:** Restaurant servings are often much larger than a typical serving size, which can contribute to overeating and difficulty managing blood glucose levels.

Incorporating American Restaurant Foods into Reverse Type 2 Diabetes Diet:

- **Choose Wisely:** Opt for dishes that are rich in vegetables, lean proteins, and whole grains. Be wary of dishes that are fried or covered in heavy sauces, as these often contain hidden sugars and unhealthy fats.
- **Mind Portion Sizes:** Be mindful of the typically large portion sizes at restaurants. Consider sharing a meal or packing half to take home.
- **Request Modifications:** Don't hesitate to request modifications to your meal to make it more diabetes-friendly. Many restaurants are willing to accommodate such requests.

* * *

The following section of this chapter presents comprehensive tables of foods that are fully compliant with Reverse Type 2 Diabetes Diet.

Each entry is accompanied by crucial information such as serving size, Glycemic Index (GI), Glycemic Load (GL), and Net Carbohydrates, enabling the reader to make informed decisions about portion sizes and meal planning.

However, it's important to note that not all compliant foods are equal. Some foods, while fitting within the parameters of the Reverse Type 2 Diabetes Diet, are more beneficial than others. For instance, foods that are minimally processed, lower in sodium, and rich in healthy fats are preferable. For these food items, even though GI, GL, and net carb data might not be the sole determinants of their suitability, their overall nutritional profile makes them excellent choices.

This distinction between different compliant foods enhances clarity and helps readers understand why certain foods are more desirable within the framework of the Reverse Type 2 Diabetes Diet. It also guides readers towards making healthier choices that align with the principles of this dietary approach and contribute to sustainable and effective diabetes management.

AMERICAN RESTAURANT FOODS

AMERICAN RESTAURANT FOOD	SERVING SIZE	GI	GL	NET CARB
Beef and Broccoli	1 cup (220g)	50	5	10g
Beef Chili	1 cup (240g)	45	6.8	15g
Beef Stew	1 cup (245g)	40	6	15g
Caesar Salad	1 salad (215g)	20	1.6	8g
Caesar Salad	1.5 cups (150g)	35	5.3	15g
Chicken Caesar Wrap	1 wrap (230g)	40	8	20g
Chicken Fajita	1 fajita (100g)	45	6.8	15g
Chicken Pot Roast	1 serving (300g)	45	6.8	15g
Chicken Tenders	3 tenders (150g)	55	8.3	15g
Cobb Salad	1 salad (200g)	20	2	10g
Crab Cakes	2 cakes (200g)	35	5.3	15g
Deviled Eggs	2 eggs (100g)	0	0	2g
Fried Catfish	1 fillet (200g)	50	7.5	15g
Fried Chicken	2 pieces (150g)	50	10	20g
Green Bean Casserole	1 cup (200g)	50	5	10g
Grilled Salmon	1 fillet (154g)	50	0	0g
Hamburger Steak	1 patty (200g)	55	2.8	5g
Lobster Bisque	1 cup (240g)	45	6.8	15g
Meatloaf	1 slice (150g)	50	5	10g
New York Strip Steak	1 steak (200g)	50	0	0g
Omelette, cheese	1 omelette (154g)	50	1.5	3g
Prime Rib	1 serving (350g)	40	0	0g
Prime Rib	6 oz (170g)	50	0	0g
Pulled Pork Sliders	1 slider (100g)	45	4.5	10g

AMERICAN RESTAURANT FOOD	SERVING SIZE	GI	GL	NET CARB
Shrimp Scampi	1 serving (300g)	50	5	10g
Smoked Brisket	1 serving (200g)	55	2.8	5g
Southern Fried Chicken	1 piece (150g)	55	5.5	10g
Texas Chili	1 cup (240g)	45	6.8	15g
Waldorf Salad	1 salad (200g)	20	3	15g

BREADS AND BAKED PRODUCTS

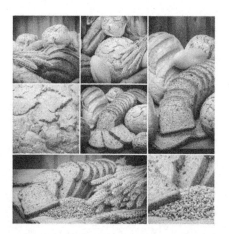

Bread and baked products are integral to many diets, including those targeted at reversing type 2 diabetes. Their role in such a diet must be considered carefully, with an emphasis on understanding their impact on glycemic load (GL) and how well they align with the objectives of the Reverse Type 2 Diabetes Diet. Knowledge of these foods' benefits and potential drawbacks allows for more informed dietary choices that bolster diabetes management and overall health.

Benefits of Breads and Baked Products:

- **Fiber-Rich**: Whole-grain bread and baked goods, including whole wheat bread, oatmeal cookies, and bran muffins, are rich sources of dietary fiber, facilitating a steady release of glucose into the bloodstream. This process helps mitigate sudden blood sugar spikes, improving glycemic control.
- **Nutrient-Dense**: Whole-grain bread and baked goods supply essential nutrients such as B-vitamins, iron, and magnesium. Compared to their refined white counterparts, these whole-grain options retain the nutrient-rich bran and germ of the grain. This nutrient density can help prevent deficiencies commonly associated with type 2 diabetes and enhance overall health.
- **Promote Satiety and Portion Control**: Whole grains and seeds in bread and baked products can enhance satiety, helping curb appetite. Incorporating these foods in moderate amounts can assist with portion control, preventing overeating, and promoting weight management, a key aspect of diabetes reversal.

Drawbacks of Breads and Baked Products:

- **High Glycemic Load**: Refined grain bread and baked goods exhibit a high glycemic load, leading to an abrupt spike in blood sugar levels. This can be problematic for individuals with type 2 diabetes. Therefore, opting for products with a lower glycemic load, like whole grain options or those made with alternative low-glycemic load flours such as almond or coconut, is advisable.
- **Added Sugars and Unhealthy Fats**: Commercially produced baked goods often contain high levels of added sugars and unhealthy fats. These elements can contribute to weight gain, increased insulin resistance, and higher blood sugar levels. It's

crucial to scrutinize labels and choose products low in added sugars and trans fats.

- **Portion Control Challenges**: Even whole-grain bread and baked goods can be calorie-dense, making overconsumption easy and potentially leading to excess calorie intake. Practicing portion control and awareness of serving sizes can help mitigate this risk.

Incorporating Breads and Baked Products into Reverse Type 2 Diabetes Diet:

To successfully include bread and baked products in your eating plan, consider the following:

- **Choose Whole Grains**: Prioritize whole grain bread, whole wheat tortillas, and other baked goods made with whole grain flour. Identify keywords like "whole wheat," "whole grain," or "100% whole" on product labels.
- **Monitor Glycemic Load**: Choose bread and baked goods with a lower glycemic load to minimize blood sugar spikes. Generally, whole grains have a lower glycemic load than refined grains.
- **Control Portion Sizes**: Avoid excessive calorie intake by keeping portions in check. Adhere to recommended serving sizes and consider using smaller plates or bowls to help maintain portion control.
- **Consider Homemade Options**: Baking at home provides the advantage of ingredient control, allowing you to reduce added sugars and unhealthy fats. Experiment with alternative flours such as almond, coconut, or whole wheat pastry flour to enhance the nutrient density and fiber content.
- **Adopt a Mediterranean Approach**: Incorporate bread and baked products with other elements of the Mediterranean diet, including vegetables, legumes, lean proteins, and healthy

fats. This diet emphasizes whole foods and can help balance the glycemic load of a meal.

* * *

The following section of this chapter presents comprehensive tables of foods that are fully compliant with Reverse Type 2 Diabetes Diet. Each entry is accompanied by crucial information such as serving size, Glycemic Index (GI), Glycemic Load (GL), and Net Carbohydrates, enabling the reader to make informed decisions about portion sizes and meal planning.

However, it's important to note that not all compliant foods are equal. Some foods, while fitting within the parameters of the Reverse Type 2 Diabetes Diet, are more beneficial than others. For instance, foods that are minimally processed, lower in sodium, and rich in healthy fats are preferable. For these food items, even though GI, GL, and net carb data might not be the sole determinants of their suitability, their overall nutritional profile makes them excellent choices.

This distinction between different compliant foods enhances clarity and helps readers understand why certain foods are more desirable within the framework of the Reverse Type 2 Diabetes Diet. It also guides readers towards making healthier choices that align with the principles of this dietary approach and contribute to sustainable and effective diabetes management.

BREADS AND BAKED PRODUCTS

FRUITS & FRUIT PRODUCTS	SERVING SIZE	GI	GL	NET CARB
LOW GLYCEMIC LOAD FOODS				
Biscotti	1 biscotti, 20g	40	8	12g
Brioche	1 slice, 30g	54	8	15g
Butter Cookies	1 cookie, 30g	50	7	11g
Cheese and Herb Biscuits	1 biscuit, 35g	62	5	13g
Coconut Macaroons	1 macaroon, 20g	50	5	10g
Drop Biscuits	1 biscuit, 30g	62	5	11g
Garlic Butter Biscuits	1 biscuit, 25g	62	3	10g
Green Onion Biscuits	1 biscuit, 28g	55	7	14g
Italian Bread	1 slice, 30g	70	10	14g
Lemon Cookies	1 cookie, 30g	55	9	14g
Pão de Queijo	1 piece, 30g	35	5	15g
Peanut Butter Blossoms	1 cookie, 30g	50	7	13g
Peanut Butter Cookies	1 cookie, 30g	50	7	13g
Pesto Biscuits	1 biscuit, 28g	65	8	15g
Pumpernickel Bread	1 slice, 30g	50	6	13g
Pumpkin Biscuits	1 biscuit, 28g	70	9	15g
Quiche	1 slice, 100g	30	3	10g
Raspberry Tart	1 slice, 100g	65	6	15g
Rosemary Biscuits	1 biscuit, 38g	62	6	15g
Rye Bread	1 slice, 25g	50	7	14g
Shortbread Cookies	1 cookie, 30g	50	7	11g
Snickerdoodle Cookies	1 cookie, 30g	55	9	14g
Sourdough Bread	1 slice, 30g	52	8	15g
Strudel	1 slice, 100g	65	6	15g

FRUITS & FRUIT PRODUCTS	SERVING SIZE	GI	GL	NET CARB
Tres Leches Cake	1 slice, 100g	25	6	10g
Whole Wheat Bread	1 cookie, 30g	60	9	14g

LEGUMES AND PULSES

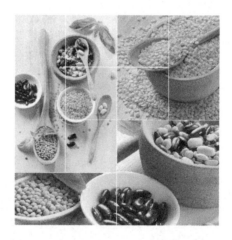

Legumes and pulses are a versatile and nutritious inclusion in many diets, playing an integral role in type 2 diabetes reversal plans. Their introduction into a diabetes reversal diet, however, requires some consideration, keeping in mind their glycemic load (GL) and compatibility with a Reverse Type 2 Diabetes Diet. By understanding the benefits and potential pitfalls of beans and their by-products, individuals can make educated decisions to bolster their diabetes management and overall well-being.

Advantages of legumes and pulses:

- **Rich in Fiber**: Beans and their by-products are renowned for their high fiber content. Dietary fiber moderates the digestion and absorption of carbohydrates, facilitating a gradual release of glucose into the bloodstream. This, in turn, helps avoid abrupt blood sugar spikes, thus enhancing glycemic control.
- **Protein-Heavy**: Beans are a great source of plant-based protein, a vital part of a diabetes-friendly diet. Unlike carbohydrates, protein doesn't significantly affect blood glucose levels and can aid in promoting feelings of fullness, thereby assisting with weight management.
- **Nutrient-Dense**: Beans contain essential nutrients such as iron, magnesium, potassium, and B vitamins. These nutrients support various bodily functions and can counteract the deficiencies often observed in individuals with type 2 diabetes.

Possible Drawbacks of Beans and By-Products:

- **Digestive Discomfort**: Beans can sometimes lead to digestive discomfort due to their high fiber content. Soaking beans before cooking and chewing them thoroughly can help alleviate these symptoms.
- **Caloric Density**: While beans are nutrient-dense, they are also relatively high in calories. Overconsumption can lead to weight gain, making portion control essential.

Incorporating Beans and By-Products into Reverse Type 2 Diabetes Diet:

Here are some tips to include beans and their by-products in your diet:

- **Choose Beans as a Protein Source**: Beans can serve as a low-fat, high-fiber alternative to meat or other animal proteins. This substitution can help maintain stable blood sugar levels.

- **Emphasize Whole Foods**: Opt for whole beans over processed bean products to limit sodium and added sugars. Canned beans are acceptable if rinsed thoroughly to remove excess salt.
- **Mind Portion Sizes**: Despite their health benefits, beans are high in calories. Practice portion control to prevent excessive calorie intake. The typical serving size for beans and their by-products is about 15-20 grams. The tables provided outline the GL, GI, and net carb content per serving, helping you make an informed choice.
- **Experiment with Bean By-Products**: Consider incorporating by-products such as tofu, tempeh, and edamame into your diet. These provide a protein-rich, low-carb alternative to other protein sources. However, avoid highly processed alternatives such as certain meat substitutes that may be high in additives and sodium.

* * *

The following section of this chapter presents comprehensive tables of foods that are fully compliant with Reverse Type 2 Diabetes Diet. Each entry is accompanied by crucial information such as serving size, Glycemic Index (GI), Glycemic Load (GL), and Net Carbohydrates, enabling the reader to make informed decisions about portion sizes and meal planning.

However, it's important to note that not all compliant foods are equal. Some foods, while fitting within the parameters of the Reverse Type 2 Diabetes Diet, are more beneficial than others. For instance, foods that are minimally processed, lower in sodium, and rich in healthy fats are preferable. For these food items, even though GI, GL, and net carb data might not be the sole determinants of their suitability, their overall nutritional profile makes them excellent choices.

This distinction between different compliant foods enhances clarity and helps readers understand why certain foods are more desirable within the framework of the Reverse Type 2 Diabetes Diet. It also guides readers towards making healthier choices that align with the principles of this dietary approach and contribute to sustainable and effective diabetes management.

LEGUMES &PULSES

	SERVING SIZE	GI	GL	NET CARB
Baby lima beans	½ cup, 100g	32	6	13g
Adzuki Bean Flour	¼ cup, 30g	32	5.8	18g
Adzuki Bean Sprout Powder	¼ cup, 30g	15	2.1	14g
Alfalfa Sprout Powder	¼ cup, 30g	15	0.8	5g
Amaranth Sprout Powder	¼ cup, 30g	35	7	20g
Azuki Bean Flour	¼ cup, 30g	33	6.2	18.9g
Barley Sprout Powder	¼ cup, 30g	25	4.5	18g
Black Bean Flour	¼ cup, 30g	30	3.2	10.5g
Black beans	½ cup, 100g	30	5	13g
Black Eyed Pea Flour	¼ cup, 30g	42	7.9	18.9g
Black turtle beans	½ cup, 100g	30	5	13g
Black-eyed peas	½ cup, 100g	41	8	19g
Broad Bean Flour (Fava Bean Flour)	¼ cup, 30g	79	13.7	17.4g
Broccoli Sprout Powder	¼ cup, 30g	15	1.2	8g
Buckwheat Sprout Powder	¼ cup, 30g	45	9	20g
Butter Bean Flour (Lima Bean Flour)	¼ cup, 30g	31	5.6	18g
Cabbage Sprout Powder	¼ cup, 30g	15	1.2	8g
Cannellini Bean Flour	¼ cup, 30g	31	5.6	18g
Cannellini beans	½ cup, 100g	31	4	13g
Chia Sprout Powder	¼ cup, 30g	15	0.6	4g
Chickpea Flour (Besan)	¼ cup, 30g	44	5.8	13.2g
Chickpeas, garbanzo beans	½ cup, 100g	28	6	16g

	SERVING SIZE	GI	GL	NET CARB
Clover Sprout Powder	¼ cup, 30g	15	0.8	5g
Cowpeas	½ cup, 100g	29	7	18g
Cranberry Bean Flour	¼ cup, 30g	29	5.2	18g
Dragon's tongue beans	½ cup, 100g	31	2	5g
Fava Bean Flour	¼ cup, 30g	79	13.7	17.4g
Fava beans	½ cup, 100g	32	7	13g
Flageolet beans	½ cup, 100g	31	4	14g
French Green Lentil Flour	¼ cup, 30g	28	5	18g
Garbanzo Bean Flour (Gram Flour)	¼ cup, 30g	28	4.9	17.4g
Garlic Sprout Powder	¼ cup, 30g	15	2.1	14g
Great Northern Bean Flour	¼ cup, 30g	36	6.5	18g
Great Northern Beans	½ cup, 100g	31	5	15g
Green Pea Flour	¼ cup, 30g	48	8.6	18g
Green peas	½ cup, 100g	68	4	9g
Kale Sprout Powder	¼ cup, 30g	15	1.2	8g
Kidney Bean Flour	¼ cup, 30g	24	4.3	18g
Kidney beans	½ cup, 100g	29	7	16g
Lentil Flour	¼ cup, 30g	29	4.4	15g
Lentil Sprout Powder	¼ cup, 30g	25	3.8	15g
Lentils	½ cup, 100g	29	5	12g
Lima bean flour	½ cup, 100g	32	4	19g
Lima Bean Flour	¼ cup, 30g	32	5.8	18g
Lima beans	½ cup, 100g	32	8	20g
Moth Bean Flour	¼ cup, 30g	29	5.5	18.9g
Mung Bean Flour	¼ cup, 30g	25	4.7	18.9g
Mung Bean Sprout Powder	¼ cup, 30g	15	1.8	12g

	SERVING SIZE	GI	GL	NET CARB
Mung beans	½ cup, 100g	32	4	12g
Navy Bean Flour	¼ cup, 30g	38	6.8	18g
Navy beans	½ cup, 100g	31-58	8	11g
Onion Sprout Powder	¼ cup, 30g	15	2.3	15g
Pea Sprout Powder	¼ cup, 30g	15	2.1	14g
Peanuts	1 oz, 28g	30-33	1	3g
Pinto Bean Flour	¼ cup, 30g	39	7	18g
Quinoa Sprout Powder	¼ cup, 30g	35	7	20g
Radish Sprout Powder	¼ cup, 30g	15	0.8	5g
Red beans	½ cup, 100g	35-58	10	15g
Red kidney beans	½ cup, 100g	24-40	7	13g
Red Lentil Flour	¼ cup, 30g	26	4.7	18g
Red lentils	½ cup, 100g	20-44	8	13g
Soy Flour	¼ cup, 30g	15	0.9	6g
Soybean Sprout Powder	¼ cup, 30g	15	1.2	8g
Soybeans	½ cup, 100g	18-33	6	10g
Split peas	½ cup, 100g	22-32	5	12g
Split peas	½ cup, 100g	22-32	5	12g
Sunflower Sprout Powder	¼ cup, 30g	15	1.2	8g
Wheatgrass Sprout Powder	¼ cup, 30g	15	2.3	15g
White Bean Flour	¼ cup, 30g	31	5.6	18g
White beans	½ cup, 100g	31-45	7	12g
Yellow Split Pea Flour	¼ cup, 30g	35	6.3	18g
Red kidney beans	½ cup, 100g	24-40	7	13g
Red Lentil Flour	¼ cup, 30g	26	4.7	18g
Red lentils	½ cup, 100g	20-44	8	13g
Soy Flour	¼ cup, 30g	15	0.9	6g
Soybean Sprout Powder	¼ cup, 30g	15	1.2	8g

	SERVING SIZE	GI	GL	NET CARB
Soybeans	½ cup, 100g	18-33	6	10g
Split peas	½ cup, 100g	22-32	5	12g
Split peas	½ cup, 100g	22-32	5	12g
Sunflower Sprout Powder	¼ cup, 30g	15	1.2	8g
Wheatgrass Sprout Powder	¼ cup, 30g	15	2.3	15g

BEVERAGES AND DRINKS

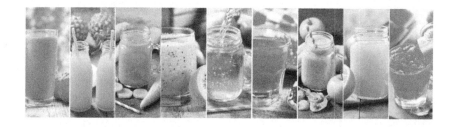

Beverages are an integral part of our diet and hydration routine, and their careful selection is paramount for those following Reverse Type 2 Diabetes Diet. Assessing the impact of different drinks on glycemic load (GL) and their alignment with Reverse Type 2 Diabetes Diet can help individuals make informed choices that support their diabetes management and overall health. Understanding the pros and cons of various beverages is crucial in making these decisions.

Advantages of Select Beverages:

- **Hydration**: Certain beverages, especially water, provide essential hydration without impacting blood glucose levels.
- **Nutrient-Rich Options**: Drinks like vegetable juice, fortified

plant-based milk, and low-fat dairy drinks can offer important nutrients. These contribute to overall health and help prevent nutrient deficiencies common in individuals with type 2 diabetes.

- **Convenient Protein Source**: When mixed with water or milk, Protein powders can provide a convenient source of protein that doesn't significantly impact blood glucose levels.

Drawbacks of Certain Beverages:

- **High Sugar Content**: Many commercial drinks, such as sodas, fruit juices, and sweetened coffees, contain high amounts of added sugars. These can lead to rapid spikes in blood sugar and contribute to weight gain, thereby counteracting efforts for diabetes reversal and weight loss.
- **Poor in Fiber**: Most beverages lack dietary fiber, a nutrient important for maintaining stable blood sugar levels and promoting satiety.
- **Artificial Sweeteners**: Some artificially sweetened or "diet" drinks can have potential negative health impacts and may trigger cravings for sweet foods.

Incorporating Beverages into Reverse Type 2 Diabetes Diet:

Here are some guidelines to consider:

- **Prioritize Water**: Water should be your go-to choice for hydration. It has a GL of zero and does not impact blood sugar levels.
- **Choose Unsweetened Beverages**: Opt for unsweetened drinks like black coffee or unsweetened tea. If you prefer flavored drinks, consider adding a slice of lemon, lime, or cucumber to your water for a low-calorie flavor boost.
- **Limit Fruit Juices**: Fruit juices can be high in sugars, rapidly

increasing blood glucose levels. Stick to small portions, or consider diluting juice with water.

- **Mindful Dairy Consumption**: Low-fat dairy drinks can be a source of essential nutrients but also contain lactose, a type of sugar. Monitoring portion sizes is key.
- **Avoid Sugary and Artificially Sweetened Drinks**: Avoid high-sugar drinks like sweetened teas, sodas, and energy drinks. Be wary of artificially sweetened beverages due to their potential negative health effects and their possible contribution to increased cravings for sweet foods.
- **Consider Protein Powders**: Opt for unsweetened protein powders, which can provide a convenient and low-GL source of protein.
- **Portion Control**: Even healthy beverages can contribute to high-calorie intake if consumed in large amounts. The provided tables list the GL, GI, and net carb content of common beverages per serving size, typically around 15-20 grams.

* * *

The following section of this chapter presents comprehensive tables of foods that are fully compliant with Reverse Type 2 Diabetes Diet. Each entry is accompanied by crucial information such as serving size, Glycemic Index (GI), Glycemic Load (GL), and Net Carbohydrates, enabling the reader to make informed decisions about portion sizes and meal planning.

However, it's important to note that not all compliant foods are equal. Some foods, while fitting within the parameters of the Reverse Type 2 Diabetes Diet, are more beneficial than others. For instance, foods that are minimally processed, lower in sodium, and rich in healthy fats are preferable. For these food items, even though GI, GL, and net carb data might not be the sole determinants of their suitability, their overall nutritional profile makes them excellent choices.

This distinction between different compliant foods enhances clarity and helps readers understand why certain foods are more desirable within the framework of the Reverse Type 2 Diabetes Diet. It also guides readers towards making healthier choices that align with the principles of this dietary approach and contribute to sustainable and effective diabetes management.

BEVERAGES & DRINKS

BEVERAGES & DRINKS	SERVING SIZE	GI	GL	NET CARB
Almond Milk	1 cup (240ml)	30	0.6	2g
Almond Milk, unsweetened	1 cup (240ml)	30	0.3	1g
Almond-Flavored Water	1 cup (240ml)	0	0	0g
Americano	1 cup (240ml)	0	0	0g
Apple Cider Vinegar (diluted as a beverage)	1 cup (240ml)	0	0	0g
Basil Infused Water	1 cup (240ml)	0	0	0g
Beer	1 cup (240ml)	50	4	8g
Beer (light)	1 cup (240ml)	50	2	4g
Beer (regular)	1 cup (240ml)	50	4	8g
Beet Kvass	1 cup (240ml)	60	6	10g
Black Tea	1 cup (240ml)	0	0	0g
Bloody Mary	1 cup (240ml)	0	0	6g
Blueberry Infused Water	1 cup (240ml)	0	0	0g
Bulletproof Coffee	1 cup (240ml)	0	0	0g
Bulletproof Coffee (with MCT oil)	1 cup (240ml)	0	0	0g
Buttermilk	1 cup (240ml)	30	3.3	11g
Café au lait	1 cup (240ml)	30	1.2	4g
Caffè Breve	1 cup (240ml)	50	2	4g
Caffè Corretto	1 cup (240ml)	0	0	0g
Cappuccino	1 cup (240ml)	50	4	8g
Carbonated Water with Natural Flavors	1 cup (240ml)	0	0	0g
Carbonated Water with Stevia and Natural Flavors	1 cup (240ml)	0	0	0g

BEVERAGES & DRINKS	SERVING SIZE	GI	GL	NET CARB
Cashew Milk	1 cup (240ml)	30	1.2	4g
Cashew Milk, unsweetened	1 cup (240ml)	35	0.7	2g
Chai Tea	1 cup (240ml)	0	0	0g
Chamomile Tea	1 cup (240ml)	0	0	0g
Cherry Infused Water	1 cup (240ml)	0	0	0g
Citrus Infused Water	1 cup (240ml)	0	0	0g
Club Soda	1 cup (240ml)	0	0	0g
Coconut Milk	1 cup (240ml)	45	2.7	6g
Coconut Milk Kefir	1 cup (240ml)	30	1.2	4g
Coconut Milk, unsweetened	1 cup (240ml)	45	0.9	2g
Coconut Water	1 cup (240ml)	35	3.2	9g
Coconut Water Kefir	1 cup (240ml)	40	2.4	6g
Coconut-Flavored Water	1 cup (240ml)	0	0	0g
Cold Brew Coffee	1 cup (240ml)	0	0	0g
Cortado	4 fl oz (120g)	0	0	0g
Cucumber Infused Water	1 cup (240ml)	0	0	0g
Diet Cola	1 cup (240ml)	0	0	0g
Diet Ginger Ale	1 cup (240ml)	0	0	0g
Diet Lemon-Lime Soda	1 cup (240ml)	0	0	0g
Diet Root Beer	1 cup (240ml)	0	0	0g
Doppio	¼ cup (60ml)	0	0	0g
Electrolyte Water	1 cup (240ml)	0	0	0g
Energy Drink (sugar-free)	1 cup (240ml)	0	0	0g
Erythritol-Sweetened Soda	1 cup (240ml)	0	0	0g
Espresso	¼ cup (60ml)	0	0	0g
Flat White	1 cup (240ml)	0	0	0g

BEVERAGES & DRINKS	SERVING SIZE	GI	GL	NET CARB
Flavored Tea	1 cup (240ml)	0	0	0g
Flax Milk	1 cup (240ml)	45	0.9	2g
Flax Milk, unsweetened	1 cup (240ml)	45	0.5	1g
Fruit Kefir	1 cup (240ml)	30	2.7	9g
Fruit Wine	5 fl oz (148g)	30	2.7	9g
Ginger Tea	1 cup (240ml)	0	0	0g
Green Tea	1 cup (240ml)	0	0	0g
Green Tea-Flavored Water	1 cup (240ml)	0	0	0g
Hazelnut Milk	1 cup (240ml)	30	1.2	4g
Hazelnut Milk, unsweetened	1 cup (240ml)	30	0.6	2g
Hemp Milk	1 cup (240ml)	30	0.6	2g
Hemp Milk, unsweetened	1 cup (240ml)	30	0.3	1g
Herbal Fermented Teas	1 cup (240ml)	0	0	0g
Herbal Infusion (e.g., Chamomile)	1 cup (240ml)	0	0	0g
Herbal Tea	1 cup (240ml)	0	0	0g
Herbal-Infused Water (like rosemary or lavender)	1 cup (240ml)	0	0	0g
Hot Apple Toddy	1 cup (240ml)	0	0	10g
Hot Coconut Milk with Cinnamon and Turmeric	1 cup (240ml)	0	0	0g
Hot Lemon Water	1 cup (240ml)	0	0	0g
Hot Tea	1 cup (240ml)	0	0	0g
Iced Coffee	1 cup (240ml)	0	0	0g
Iced Coffee with Milk	1 cup (240ml)	0	0	0g
Iced Matcha Green Tea Latte	1 cup (240ml)	0	0	0g
Iced Tea	1 cup (240ml)	0	0	0g
Isotonic Beverage	1 cup (240ml)	50	5	10g

BEVERAGES & DRINKS	SERVING SIZE	GI	GL	NET CARB
Jun Tea	1 cup (240ml)	20	1	5g
Kefir	1 cup (240ml)	30	1.2	4g
Kiwi Infused Water	1 cup (240ml)	0	0	0g
Kombucha	1 cup (240ml)	10	0.2	2g
Kvass	1 cup (240ml)	40	3	7g
Laban Ayran	1 cup (240ml)	30	1.2	4g
Lactose-Free Protein Drink	1 cup (240ml)	30	0.9	3g
Lassi Low-carb Drink	1 cup (240ml)	30	3	10g
Latte	1 cup (240ml)	40	4	10g
Latte Macchiato	1 cup (240ml)	40	4	10g
Lemon Infused Water	1 cup (240ml)	0	0	0g
London Fog (Earl Grey Tea Latte)	1 cup (240ml)	0	0	0g
Low-Calorie Energy Drink	1 cup (240ml)	0	0	0g
Low-Calorie Fruit-Flavored Carbonated Drink	1 cup (240ml)	50	5	10g
Low-Calorie Tonic Water	1 cup (240ml)	50	5	10g
Macadamia Milk	1 cup (240ml)	35	1.1	3g
Macadamia Milk, unsweetened	1 cup (240ml)	35	0.7	2g
Macchiato	1 cup (240ml)	40	4	10g
Mango-Flavored Water	1 cup (240ml)	0	0	0g
Margarita	1 cup (240ml)	0	0	0g
Masala Chai	1 cup (240ml)	30	3	10g
Matcha Latte	1 cup (240ml)	0	0	0g
Matcha Tea	1 cup (240ml)	0	0	0g
Mead	1 cup (240ml)	10	2	20g
Milk (2%)	1 cup (240ml)	30	3.6	12g
Milk (skimmed)	1 cup (240ml)	30	3.6	12g

BEVERAGES & DRINKS	SERVING SIZE	GI	GL	NET CARB
Milk (whole)	1 cup (240ml)	30	3.6	12g
Milk Kefir	1 cup (240ml)	30	1.2	4g
Mint and Lime-Flavored Water	1 cup (240ml)	0	0	0g
Mint Infused Water	1 cup (240ml)	0	0	0g
Mint Tea	1 cup (240ml)	0	0	0g
Monk Fruit unsweetened Soda	1 cup (240ml)	0	0	0g
Moroccan Mint Tea, Unsweetened	1 cup (240ml)	0	0	0g
Mulled Wine	5 fl oz (148g)	50	7.5	15g
Oolong Tea	1 cup (240ml)	0	0	0g
Pea Protein Milk	1 cup (240ml)	30	0.6	2g
Pea Protein Milk, sweetened	1 cup (240ml)	30	4.2	14g
Pea Protein Milk, unsweetened	1 cup (240ml)	30	0.3	1g
Peach-Flavored Water	1 cup (240ml)	0	0	0g
Pineapple Infused Water	1 cup (240ml)	0	0	0g
Pistachio Milk	1 cup (240ml)	35	1.8	5g
Pistachio Milk, sweetened	1 cup (240ml)	60	9	15g
Pistachio Milk, unsweetened	1 cup (240ml)	25	0.8	3g
Pomegranate Infused Water	1 cup (240ml)	0	0	0g
Protein Shake	1 cup (240ml)	25	1.3	5g
Protein Shake (Whey Based)	1 cup (240ml)	30	2.1	7g
Quinoa Milk	1 cup (240ml)	35	1.8	5g
Quinoa Milk, unsweetened	1 cup (240ml)	25	0.8	3g
Raspberry Infused Water	1 cup (240ml)	0	0	0g

BEVERAGES & DRINKS	SERVING SIZE	GI	GL	NET CARB
Rice Wine	5 fl oz (100g)	10	0.3	3g
Ristretto	1 fl oz (30g)	0	0	0g
Rooibos Tea	1 cup (240ml)	0	0	0g
Rum	1 fl oz (30g)	0	0	0g
Sake	5 fl oz (100g)	20	0.2	1g
Seltzer Water	1 cup (240ml)	0	0	0g
Shrub (drinking vinegar)	1 cup (240ml)	0	0	0g
Soy Milk	1 cup (240ml)	30	2.4	8g
Soy Milk, unsweetened	1 cup (240ml)	20	0.8	4g
Sparkling Iced Tea (unsweetened)	1 cup (240ml)	0	0	0g
Sparkling Water	1 cup (240ml)	0	0	0g
Sports Drink (low-carb)	1 cup (240ml)	0	0	0g
Stevia-Sweetened Soda	1 cup (240ml)	0	0	0g
Strawberry Infused Water	1 cup (240ml)	0	0	0g
Sugar-Free Cream Soda	1 cup (240ml)	0	0	0g
Sugar-Free Energy Drink	1 cup (240ml)	0	0	0g
Sugar-Free Tonic Water	1 cup (240ml)	0	0	0g
Switchel	1 cup (240ml)	25	2.5	10g
Tequila	1 fl oz (30g)	0	0	0g
Tiger Nut Milk	1 cup (240ml)	45	3.6	8g
Tiger Nut Milk, unsweetened	1 cup (240ml)	30	0.3	1g
Turmeric Latte	1 cup (240ml)	40	5.6	14g
Turmeric Tea	1 cup (240ml)	0	0	0g
Vanilla-Flavored Water	1 cup (240ml)	0	0	0g
Vienna Coffee	1 cup (240ml)	0	0	0g
Vinegar (diluted as a beverage)	1 cup (240ml)	0	0	0g

BEVERAGES & DRINKS	SERVING SIZE	GI	GL	NET CARB
Vitamin-Enriched Water	1 cup (240ml)	0	0	0g
Vodka	1 fl oz (30g)	0	0	0g
Walnut Milk, unsweetened	1 cup (240ml)	25	0.3	1g
Water Kefir	1 cup (240ml)	30	1.5	5g
Water with Natural Fruit Flavors	1 cup (240ml)	0	0	0g
Whiskey	1 fl oz (30g)	0	0	0g
White Tea	1 cup (240ml)	0	0	0g
Wine	5 fl oz (148g)	0	0	0g
Wine (red)	5 fl oz (148g)	0	0	0g
Wine (white)	5 fl oz (148g)	0	0	0g
Yakult	2.7 fl oz (80g)	50	6	12g
Zero Calorie Energy Drink	1 cup (240ml)	0	0	0g
Zero Sugar Cola	1 cup (240ml)	0	0	0g
Zero Sugar Ginger Ale	1 cup (240ml)	0	0	0g
MEDIUM GLYCEMIC LOAD FOODS (consider reducing the serving size to stay below 15 grams of net carbs)				
Caffè Mocha	1 cup (240ml)	50	16	32g
Caramel Latte	1 cup (240ml)	50	12.5	25g
Caramel Macchiato	1 cup (240ml)	50	12.5	25g
Chocolate Milk	1 cup (240ml)	60	13.8	23g
Coconut Milk, sweetened	1 cup (240ml)	50	10.5	21g
Hot Mocha	1 cup (240ml)	50	15	30g
Hot Peppermint Mocha	1 cup (240ml)	50	15	30g
Iced Chai Tea Latte	1 cup (240ml)	50	12.5	25g
Malt Drink	1 cup (240ml)	50	17.5	35g
Oat Milk	1 cup (240ml)	69	16.6	24g
Post-workout Recovery Drink	1 cup (240ml)	50	12.5	25g

BEVERAGES & DRINKS	SERVING SIZE	GI	GL	NET CARB
Pre-workout Energy Drink	1 cup (240ml)	65	19.5	30g
Rice Milk, unsweetened	1 cup (240ml)	75	11.3	15g
Sarsaparilla	1 cup (240ml)	50	12.5	25g
Sports Drinks	1 cup (240ml)	60	18	30g
Tepache	1 cup (240ml)	55	13.8	25g
Thai Iced Tea	1 cup (240ml)	50	12.5	25g
Tiger Nut Milk, sweetened	1 cup (240ml)	65	15.6	24g
Tonic Water	1 cup (240ml)	50	12.5	25g
Yogurt Smoothie	1 cup (240ml)	50	15	30g

DAIRY AND PLANT-BASED ALTERNATIVES

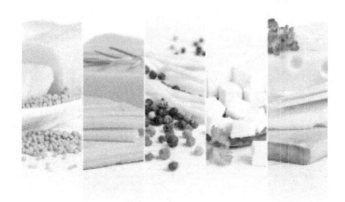

Dairy products are often a significant part of many diets, including those followed by individuals aiming to reverse type 2 diabetes. When incorporating dairy into such a diet, it's vital to assess their glycemic load (GL) and alignment with Reverse Type 2 Diabetes Diet's principles. Knowledge of the advantages and potential drawbacks of dairy aids in making informed decisions that support diabetes management and overall health.

Benefits of Dairy:

- **Rich in Nutrients**: Dairy products like cheese provide essential nutrients like calcium, protein, and, in some cases, vitamin D. These nutrients support overall health and help prevent deficiencies common in people with type 2 diabetes. For instance, a 1 oz (28 grams) serving of cheese is nutrient-dense, supplying vital nutrients while fitting well into a diabetes reversal diet.
- **Source of Probiotics**: Fermented dairy products like yogurt and kefir contain probiotics, beneficial bacteria that support gut health and may contribute to better glycemic control.

Drawbacks of Dairy:

- **Lactose Content**: Dairy products contain lactose, a sugar that can raise blood glucose levels. Additionally, individuals with lactose intolerance may struggle with consuming dairy.
- **High in Saturated Fats**: Certain dairy products, especially full-fat varieties, can be high in saturated fats. Although the health impact of saturated fats is complex, excessive intake can contribute to weight gain and heart disease risk. However, recent research suggests that dairy-derived saturated fats may not be as harmful as once thought, unlike saturated fats from other sources. Yet, it's best to consume them moderately as part of a balanced diet.
- **Potential for Processed Products**: Highly processed dairy products, such as certain types of cheese or flavored yogurts, can contain high amounts of added sugars and sodium.

Incorporating Dairy into Reverse Type 2 Diabetes Diet:

Here are some guidelines to consider:

- **Choose Low-Fat Varieties**: If necessary, opt for low-fat versions of dairy products to manage your intake of saturated fats.
- **Monitor Portion Sizes**: Maintain portion control, especially considering the calorie content of many dairy products. Even healthy dairy products can lead to weight gain if consumed excessively.
- **Limit Processed Dairy**: Avoid highly processed dairy products, which can be high in added sugars and sodium. In our "Go-To Guide: Best Foods for Reverse Type 2 Diabetes Diet," cheeses high in sodium have been removed, ensuring the recommended options align with your health goals.
- **Consider Fermented Dairy**: Include fermented dairy products like plain yogurt and kefir into your diet for their probiotic benefits.
- **Check for Added Sugars**: Read labels carefully to detect any added sugars, particularly in products like flavored yogurts and processed cheeses.

* * *

The following section of this chapter presents comprehensive tables of foods that are fully compliant with Reverse Type 2 Diabetes Diet. Each entry is accompanied by crucial information such as serving size, Glycemic Index (GI), Glycemic Load (GL), and Net Carbohydrates, enabling the reader to make informed decisions about portion sizes and meal planning.

However, it's important to note that not all compliant foods are equal. Some foods, while fitting within the parameters of the Reverse Type 2 Diabetes Diet, are more beneficial than others. For instance, foods that are minimally processed, lower in sodium, and rich in healthy fats are preferable. For these food items, even though GI, GL, and net carb data might not be the sole determinants of their suitability, their overall nutritional profile makes them excellent choices.

This distinction between different compliant foods enhances clarity and helps readers understand why certain foods are more desirable within the framework of the Reverse Type 2 Diabetes Diet. It also guides readers towards making healthier choices that align with the principles of this dietary approach and contribute to sustainable and effective diabetes management.

DAIRY & PLANT-BASED ALTERNATIVES

DAIRY & PLANT-BASED ALTERNATIVES	SERVING SIZE	GI	GL	NET CARB
LOW GLYCEMIC LOAD FOODS				
1% milk,	1 cup, 244g	27-45	5	12g
2% Greek Yogurt	1 cup, 227g	11	4	10g
2% milk	1 cup, 244g	27-45	5	12g
Almond milk yogurt	1 container (150g)	<1	<1	4g
Almond milk	1 cup, 240 ml	<1	<1	1g
American Cheese	1 oz, 28g	0	0	2g
Appenzeller	1 oz, 28g	<1	<1	0.1g
Asiago Cheese	1 oz, 28g	0	0	0g
Brie Cheese	1 oz, 28g	0	0	1g
Burrata,	1 oz, 28g	<1	<1	1g
Butter	1 tbsp, 14g	0	0	0g
Buttermilk	1 cup, 245g	46	8	12g
Camembert Cheese	1 oz, 28g	0	0	0g
Cashew milk yogurt,	1 container (150g)	<1	<1	7g
Cashew milk,	1 cup, 240 ml	<1	<1	2g
Cheddar	1 oz, 28g	<1	<1	0.4g
Chèvre	1 oz, 28g	<1	<1	0.2g
Coconut milk yogurt,	1 container (150g)	<1	<1	5g
Coconut milk,	1 cup, 240 ml	<1	<1	2g
Colby Cheese	1 oz, 28g	0	0	0g
Colby Jack Cheese	1 oz, 28g	0	0	1g
Comté	1 oz, 28g	<1	<1	0.4g

DAIRY & PLANT-BASED ALTERNATIVES	SERVING SIZE	GI	GL	NET CARB
Cottage Cheese	1 cup, 226g	10	1	6g
Cottage Cheese (Flavored)	1 cup, 226g	10	2	15g
Cottage Cheese (Large Curd)	1 cup, 240g	10	2	10g
Cottage Cheese (Low-fat)	1 cup, 226g	10	1	6g
Cottage Cheese (Non-fat)	1 cup, 226g	10	1	10g
Cottage Cheese (Small Curd)	1 cup, 240g	10	2	10g
Cream Cheese	1 oz, 28g	0	0	1g
Cream Cheese (Flavored)	1 oz, 28g	0	0	2g
Cream Cheese (Low-fat)	1 oz, 28g	0	0	1g
Cream Cheese (Non-fat)	1 oz, 28g	0	0	2g
Cream Cheese Spread	1 tbsp, 14g	0	0	1g
Creamer (Dairy-based)	1 tbsp, 15ml	47	1	5g
Creamer (Non-dairy)	1 tbsp, 15ml	34	1	4g
Edam Cheese	1 oz, 28g	0	0	1g
Emmental	1 oz, 28g	<1	<1	0.4g
Extra Firm Tofu	1/2 cup, 126g	15	0	2g
Farmer Cheese	1 cup, 226g	10	2	10g
Firm Tofu	1/2 cup, 126g	15	0	2g
Flax milk,	1 cup, 240 ml	<1	<1	1g
Fontina Cheese	1 oz, 28g	0	0	0g
Fontina,	1 oz, 28g	<1	<1	0.4g
Ghee (Clarified Butter)	1 tbsp, 14g	0	0	0g
Goat Cheese	1 oz, 28g	0	0	1g
Gouda Cheese	1 oz, 28g	0	0	1g
Greek Yogurt (Full-fat)	1 cup, 227g	11	5	10g
Greek Yogurt (Low-fat)	1 cup, 227g	11	4	10g
Greek Yogurt (Non-fat)	1 cup, 227g	11	3	10g

DAIRY & PLANT-BASED ALTERNATIVES	SERVING SIZE	GI	GL	NET CARB
Greek Yogurt (Plain)	1 cup, 227g	11	5	10g
Gruyere Cheese	1 oz, 28g	0	0	0g
Gruyere,	1 oz, 28g	<1	<1	0g
Half and Half	1 tbsp, 15ml	0	0	0g
Havarti Cheese	1 oz, 28g	0	0	1g
Hazelnut milk,	1 cup, 240 ml	<1	<1	2g
Heavy Cream	1 tbsp, 15ml	0	0	0g
Hemp milk,	1 cup, 240 ml	<1	<1	2g
Kefir	1 cup, 240g	20	4	12g
Labneh	1 oz, 28g	0	0	2g
Lactose-free milk,	1 cup, 244g	27-45	5	12g
Limburger Cheese	1 oz, 28g	0	0	0g
Manchego,	1 oz, 28g	<1	<1	0g
Mascarpone	1 oz, 28g	0	0	1g
Monterey Jack Cheese	1 oz, 28g	0	0	1g
Monterey Jack with Jalapeño,	1 oz, 28g	<1	<1	0.4g
Monterey Jack,	1 oz, 28g	<1	<1	0.5g
Mozzarella Cheese	1 oz, 28g	0	0	1g
Muenster Cheese	1 oz, 28g	0	0	0g
Neufchâtel Cheese	1 oz, 28g	0	0	1g
Non-fat Greek Yogurt	1 cup, 227g	11	3	10g
Organic milk,	1 cup, 244g	27-45	5	12g
Panela Cheese	1 oz, 28g	0	0	0g
Pea milk,	1 cup (240 ml)	34	2	2g
Pepper Jack Cheese	1 oz, 28g	0	0	1g
Provolone Cheese	1 oz, 28g	0	0	1g
Provolone piccante,	1 oz, 28g	<1	<1	0.6g
Quark	1 cup, 225g	0	0	9g

DAIRY & PLANT-BASED ALTERNATIVES	SERVING SIZE	GI	GL	NET CARB
Queso Blanco	1 oz, 28g	0	0	0g
Queso de Bola	1 oz, 28g	0	0	0g
Queso Fresco	1 oz, 28g	0	0	0g
Ricotta Cheese	1 cup, 246g	0	0	7g
Ricotta Cheese (Part-skim)	1 cup, 246g	0	0	7g
Ricotta Cheese (Whole-milk)	1 cup, 246g	0	0	11g
Ricotta,	1/4 cup, 62g	<1	<1	3g
Silken Tofu	1/2 cup, 126g	15	0	1g
Skim milk,	1 cup, 244g	27-45	4	12g
Sour Cream	1 cup, 230g	14	3	10g
Sour Cream (Low-fat)	1 cup, 230g	14	3	10g
Sour Cream (Non-fat)	1 cup, 230g	14	3	15g
Soy Butter	1 tbsp, 14g	0	0	0g
Soy Cheese	1 oz, 28g	14	0	0g
Soy Cottage Cheese	1 cup, 240g	15	3	5g
Soy Cream Cheese	1 oz, 28g	14	0	0g
Soy Creamer	1 tbsp, 15ml	34	1	2g
Soy Milk (Plain)	1 cup, 240ml	34	4	4g
Soy Milk (Unsweetened)	1 cup, 240ml	34	0	1g
Soy Milk (Vanilla)	1 cup, 240ml	34	7	10g
Soy milk,	1 cup, 240 ml	34	4	4g
Soy Protein Powder	1 scoop, 30g	25	6	2g
Soy Ricotta Cheese	1 cup, 246g	15	1	4g
Soy Sour Cream	1 tbsp, 14g	18	1	2g
Soy Whipped Topping	1 tbsp, 5g	0	0	0g
Soy Yogurt (Plain)	1 cup, 245g	32	9	15g
Soy yogurt	1 container (150g)	43	4	6g

DAIRY & PLANT-BASED ALTERNATIVES	SERVING SIZE	GI	GL	NET CARB
Soy-based Coffee Creamer	1 tbsp, 15ml	34	1	2g
Soy-based Creamer (Flavored)	1 tbsp, 15ml	34	1	2g
Soy-based Creamer (Non-dairy)	1 tbsp, 15ml	34	1	2g
Soy-based Desserts	1 serving, 100g	34	10	15g
Soy-based Milkshake	1 cup, 240ml	34	9	15g
Soy-based Whipped Cream	1 tbsp, 5g	0	0	0g
Swiss Cheese	1 oz, 28g	0	0	1g
Swiss Cheese (Flavored)	1 oz, 28g	0	0	2g
Swiss Cheese (Low-fat)	1 oz, 28g	0	0	1g
Swiss Cheese (Non-fat)	1 oz, 28g	0	0	2g
Taleggio	1 oz, 28g	<1	<1	0.1g
Tempeh	1 cup, 166g	35	5	10g
Tofu	1/2 cup, 126g	15	0	1g
Whipped Butter	1 tbsp, 14g	0	0	0g
Whipped Cream	1 cup, 240g	0	0	10g
Whipped Topping	1 cup, 76g	0	0	5g
Whipped Topping (Light)	1 cup, 120g	0	0	10g
Whole Milk Greek Yogurt	1 cup, 227g	11	5	10g
Whole milk,	1 cup (244g	27-45	5	12g
Yogurt (Greek, Low-fat)	1 cup, 245g	11	5	10g
Yogurt (Greek, Non-fat)	1 cup, 245g	11	4	10g
Yogurt (Greek, Plain)	1 cup, 245g	11	5	10g
MEDIUM GLYCEMIC LOAD FOODS (consider reducing the serving size to stay below 15 grams of net carbs)				
Frozen Yogurt	1 cup, 159g	36	11	23g
Greek Yogurt (Flavored)	1 cup, 227g	24	12	30g
Ice Cream	1 cup, 132g	51	16	28g

DAIRY & PLANT-BASED ALTERNATIVES	SERVING SIZE	GI	GL	NET CARB
Oat milk yogurt,	1 container (150g)	59	13	17g
Oat milk,	1 cup, 240 ml	70	12	24g
Quinoa milk,	1 cup, 240 ml	53	12	18g
Skim Milk Powder	1 cup, 68g	32	14	35g
Soy Ice Cream	1 cup, 132g	50	15	20g
Soy Milk (Chocolate)	1 cup, 240ml	34	12	20g
Soy Pudding	1 cup, 113g	25	13	20g
Soy Yogurt (Vanilla)	1 cup, 245g	32	12	20g
Yogurt (Greek, Flavored)	1 cup, 245g	24	12	30g
Yogurt (Low-fat)	1 cup, 245g	33	11	20g
Yogurt (Non-fat)	1 cup, 245g	33	11	25g
Yogurt (Plain)	1 cup, 245g	33	11	20g
Yogurt Drink	1 bottle, 240g	41	13	22g

DIPS AND DRESSINGS

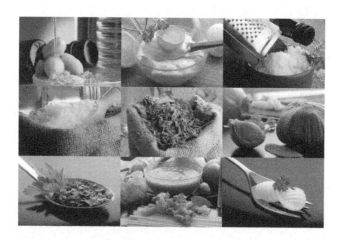

Dips and dressings can play a crucial role in a balanced diet, adding flavor and enjoyment to various dishes. However, for those following Reverse Type 2 Diabetes Diet, it's vital to be selective in choosing the right dips and dressings, focusing on those that align with the principles of low glycemic load (GL), Mediterranean Diet, the 2020-2025 Dietary Guidelines for Americans, and the twin cycle hypothesis.

There are numerous benefits to incorporating suitable dips and dressings into your diet:

- **Flavor Enhancer**: Dips and dressings can significantly boost the flavor profile of meals, making nutrient-dense foods more appealing and enjoyable.
- **Nutrient Intake**: Many dips and dressings, particularly those based on healthy fats like avocados and olive oil or nutrient-rich foods like yogurt, can provide additional nutrition, including beneficial fats, vitamins, and minerals.

However, some dips and dressings may pose potential drawbacks:

- **High Sodium Content**: Many commercially prepared dips and dressings are high in sodium, which can contribute to high blood pressure if consumed excessively.
- **High Fat Content**: Creamy or cheese-based dips and dressings can be high in fat, particularly saturated fat, which can negatively impact heart health if consumed in large quantities.
- **High Glycemic Impact**: Dips and dressings containing added sugars or made from high-GI foods can raise blood glucose levels.

When incorporating dips and dressings into your Reverse Type 2 Diabetes Diet:

- **Check the Labels**: Always read the nutrition facts and ingredient list on dips and dressings. Opt for products low in sodium, sugar, and unhealthy fats.
- **Portion Control**: Even healthy dips and dressings can contribute significant calories and fat if overconsumed. Stick to the recommended serving size, starting small and adding more as needed.
- **Make Your Own**: Homemade dips and dressings allow for

complete control over the ingredients and can often be more nutritious and less processed than store-bought versions.

* * *

The following section of this chapter presents comprehensive tables of foods that are fully compliant with Reverse Type 2 Diabetes Diet. Each entry is accompanied by crucial information such as serving size, Glycemic Index (GI), Glycemic Load (GL), and Net Carbohydrates, enabling the reader to make informed decisions about portion sizes and meal planning.

However, it's important to note that not all compliant foods are equal. Some foods, while fitting within the parameters of the Reverse Type 2 Diabetes Diet, are more beneficial than others. For instance, foods that are minimally processed, lower in sodium, and rich in healthy fats are preferable. For these food items, even though GI, GL, and net carb data might not be the sole determinants of their suitability, their overall nutritional profile makes them excellent choices.

This distinction between different compliant foods enhances clarity and helps readers understand why certain foods are more desirable within the framework of the Reverse Type 2 Diabetes Diet. It also guides readers towards making healthier choices that align with the principles of this dietary approach and contribute to sustainable and effective diabetes management.

DRESSINGS & DIPS

DRESSING & DIPS	SERVING SIZE	GI	GL	NET CARB
Artichoke Dip	1 tbsp, 15 ml	40-45	1	2.2g
Asian Sesame Dressing	2 tbsp, 30 mL	30-45	1.4	3g
Avocado Lime Dressing	2 tbsp, 30 mL	30-45	0.4	1g
Avocado Ranch Dressing	2 tbsp, 30 mL	45-50	1	2g
Baba Ghanoush	2 tbsp, 30g	40-50	1	2g
Bacon Ranch Dip	1 tbsp, 15 ml	25-30	0.4	1g
Balsamic Vinaigrette	2 tbsp, 30 mL	50-55	1.1	2g
Black Bean Dip	2 tbsp, 30g	30-35	1.2	3g
Blue Cheese Dressing	1 tbsp, 15 mL	45-50	0.5	1g
Buffalo Cauliflower Dip	1 tbsp, 15 ml	35-40	0.8	2g
Buffalo Chicken Dip	2 tbsp, 30g	30-35	0.7	2g
Caesar Dressing	2 tbsp, 30 mL	45-50	1	1g
Champagne Vinaigrette	2 tbsp, 30 mL	40-50	1	2g
Cheese Dip	1 tbsp, 15 ml	30-35	0.3	1g
Chimichurri Sauce	2 tbsp, 30 mL	30-45	0.5	1g
Chipotle Lime Dressing	2 tbsp, 30 mL	30-45	0.5	1g
Cilantro Lime Dip	1 tbsp, 15 ml	25-30	0.3	1g
Clam Dip	1 tbsp, 15 ml	25-30	0.3	1g
Corn Dip	1 tbsp, 15 ml	55-60	2.5	4.2g
Creamy Garlic Dressing	2 tbsp, 30 mL	30-45	0.5	1g
Creamy Italian Dressing	2 tbsp, 30 mL	30-45	0.5	1g
Creamy Ranch Dressing	2 tbsp, 30 mL	30-45	0.5	1g
Cucumber Dill Dressing	2 tbsp, 30 mL	30-45	0.5	1g
Cucumber Dip	1 tbsp, 15 ml	20-25	0.2	0.8g

DRESSING & DIPS	SERVING SIZE	GI	GL	NET CARB
Deviled Egg Dip	1 tbsp, 15 ml	20-25	0.1	0.5g
Edamame Dip	1 tbsp, 15 ml	20-25	0.3	1.2g
Fava Bean Dip	1 tbsp, 15 ml	30-40	0.8	2g
Feta Dip	1 tbsp, 15 ml	20-25	0.1	0.5g
Ginger Soy Dip	1 tbsp, 15 ml	25-30	0.3	1g
Gochujang Dressing	1 tbsp, 15 mL	30-45	0.5	1g
Gouda Dip	1 tbsp, 15 ml	20-25	0.1	0.5g
Greek Yogurt Dip	1 tbsp, 15 ml	25-30	0.3	1.2g
Green Goddess Dip	1 tbsp, 15 ml	20-25	0.3	1g
Hoisin Dip	1 tbsp, 15 ml	40-50	1.1	2.2g
Horseradish Dip	1 tbsp, 15 ml	25-30	0.3	1g
Hot Crab Dip	1 tbsp, 15 ml	20-25	0.1	0.7g
Hummus	2 tbsp, 30g	30-35	1.4	4g
Italian Dressing	1 tbsp, 15 mL	30-50	0.5	1g
Jalapeño Popper Dip	2 tbsp, 30g	30-35	0.7	2g
Lemon Vinaigrette	2 tbsp, 30 mL	30-45	0.4	1g
Mango Chutney Dip	1 tbsp, 15 ml	40-50	1.5	3g
Mango Salsa	1 tbsp, 15 ml	40-50	1.5	3g
Mexican Street Corn Dip	1 tbsp, 15 ml	55-60	2.1	4g
Mustard Dip	1 tbsp, 15 ml	20-25	0.1	0.8g
Nacho Dip	1 tbsp, 15 ml	30-35	0.5	1.2g
Olive Tapenade	1 tbsp, 15 ml	15-20	0.2	0.8g
Onion Dip	1 tbsp, 15 ml	25-30	0.4	1g
Peanut Butter Dip	1 tbsp, 15 ml	40-55	1.2	2.2g
Pesto Dip	1 tbsp, 15 ml	20-30	0.3	1g
Pico de Gallo	2 tbsp, 30g	20-25	0.5	2g
Pineapple Salsa	1 tbsp, 15 ml	40-55	1.5	3g
Roasted Eggplant Dip	1 tbsp, 15 ml	30-45	0.8	1.5g

DRESSING & DIPS	SERVING SIZE	GI	GL	NET CARB
Roasted Garlic Dip	1 tbsp, 15 ml	30-40	0.8	1.5g
Roasted Red Pepper Dip	1 tbsp, 15 ml	35-40	0.9	2g
Roasted Tomato Dip	1 tbsp, 15 ml	30-35	0.5	1.2g
Roquefort Cheese Dressing	2 tbsp, 30 mL	40-50	0.5	2g
Salmon Dip	1 tbsp, 15 ml	20-25	0.1	0.5g
Shrimp Dip	1 tbsp, 15 ml	20-25	0.1	0.5g
Smoked Gouda Dip	1 tbsp, 15 ml	20-25	0.1	0.5g
Smoked Salmon Dip	1 tbsp, 15 ml	20-25	0.1	0.5g
Smoky Red Pepper Dip	1 tbsp, 15 ml	35-40	0.9	2g
Southwestern Dip	1 tbsp, 15 ml	30-40	0.8	1.5g
Spicy Pimiento Cheese Dip	1 tbsp, 15 ml	35-50	0.9	1.5g
Sweet Potato Dip	1 tbsp, 15 ml	50-55	1.6	3g
Tapenade	1 tbsp, 15 ml	15-20	0.1	0.8g
Teriyaki Dip	1 tbsp, 15 ml	40-55	1.2	2.2g
Tex-Mex Dip	1 tbsp, 15 ml	30-45	0.8	1.5g
Thai Peanut Dip	1 tbsp, 15 ml	40-55	0.6	2.2g
Tomato Basil Dip	1 tbsp, 15 ml	25-30	0.3	1g
Tuna Dip	1 tbsp, 15 ml	20-25	0.1	0.5g
Wasabi Dip	1 tbsp, 15 ml	20-25	0.1	0.5g
Whipped Feta Dip	1 tbsp, 15 ml	20-25	0.1	0.5g
Whipped Goat Cheese Dip	1 tbsp, 15 ml	20-25	0.1	0.5g
White Queso Dip	1 tbsp, 15 ml	30-35	0.4	1g
Zucchini Dip	1 tbsp, 15 ml	20-25	0.2	1g

GRAINS, CEREALS AND PASTA

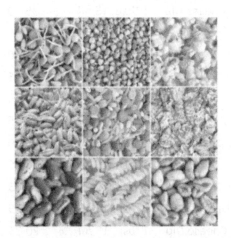

Grains and cereals form a major part of many diets globally, including those of individuals pursuing Reverse Type 2 Diabetes Diet. To evaluate their inclusion, it's essential to assess their glycemic load (GL), nutritional content, and their fit with Reverse Type 2 Diabetes Diet. Grasping the benefits and potential drawbacks of grains and cereals can enable individuals to make informed dietary choices that aid diabetes management and overall health.

Benefits of Grains and Cereals:

- **Nutrient-Dense:** Whole grains and cereals contain essential nutrients, such as dietary fiber, B vitamins, and minerals like iron, magnesium, and selenium.
- **Source of Fiber:** Whole grains are a fantastic source of dietary fiber, which can delay sugar absorption into your bloodstream and prevent abrupt increases in glucose and insulin levels.

Potential Drawbacks of Grains and Cereals:

- **Refined Grains:** Refined grains, like white rice and white bread, have been stripped of their fiber-rich outer layers, leaving predominantly the starchy endosperm. This could lead to rapid surges in blood sugar levels.
- **High in Carbohydrates:** Grains and cereals are carbohydrate-rich, which can elevate blood sugar levels if not appropriately portioned.

Incorporating Grains and Cereals into Reverse Type 2 Diabetes Diet:

- **Opt for Whole Grains:** Choose whole grains and cereals over their refined alternatives. Nutritious whole grains like brown rice, oatmeal, quinoa, and whole-grain bread or pasta have a lower GL.
- **Monitor Portion Sizes:** As grains and cereals are carbohydrate-rich, monitoring portion sizes can aid blood sugar level management and facilitate weight loss.
- **Read Labels Diligently:** Pay careful attention to labels when purchasing grain or cereal products. Look for products and by-products that list whole grains as primary ingredients, and avoid those with added sugars.

* * *

The following section of this chapter presents comprehensive tables of foods that are fully compliant with Reverse Type 2 Diabetes Diet. Each entry is accompanied by crucial information such as serving size, Glycemic Index (GI), Glycemic Load (GL), and Net Carbohydrates, enabling the reader to make informed decisions about portion sizes and meal planning.

However, it's important to note that not all compliant foods are equal. Some foods, while fitting within the parameters of the Reverse Type 2 Diabetes Diet, are more beneficial than others. For instance, foods that are minimally processed, lower in sodium, and rich in healthy fats are preferable. For these food items, even though GI, GL, and net carb data might not be the sole determinants of their suitability, their overall nutritional profile makes them excellent choices.

GRAINS, CEREALS & PASTA

GRAINS, CEREALS & PASTA	SERVING SIZE	GI	GL	NET CARB
LOW GLYCEMIC LOAD FOODS *consider reducing when necessary the serving size to stay below 15 grams of net carbs*				
Amaranth	½ cup cooked, 123g	35	3.5	10g
Barley	½ cup cooked, 89g	28	4.5	16g
Barley Hulled	½ cup cooked, 89g	25-30	5.5	20g
Bhutanese Red Rice	½ cup cooked, 92g	45	9.4	19.2g
Black Rice	½ cup cooked, 93g	44	9.7	16g
Brown Rice Porridge	½ cup cooked, 98g	55-70	7.5	16g
Buckwheat	½ cup cooked, 84g	45-55	7.5	16.5g
Buckwheat Groats	½ cup cooked, 84g	45	6.5	14.5g
Buckwheat Noodles	½ cup cooked, 57g	45	9.5	21g
Buckwheat Porridge	½ cup cooked, 84g	50-65	7	11.5g
Buckwheat Spaghetti	½ cup cooked, 70g	45	9.5	21g
Bulgur	½ cup cooked, 91g	46	6	13g
Canned Hominy	½ cup, 82g	40-45	6	12g
Corn Bran Crude	½ cup, 30g	40-45	4.5	9.5g
Eggplant Lasagna	½ cup, 1200g	50	5	10g
Four Cheese Lasagna	½ cup, 120g	50	4	10g
Freekeh	½ cup cooked, 81g	43	6	14g
Grits	½ cup cooked, 121g	60-80	7.5	14g
Hominy Canned Yellow	½ cup, 82g	40-45	6	12g
Hulled Barley	½ cup cooked, 78g	28	4.5	16g
Japanese Somen	½ cup, 73g	45-50	9.5	19g
Kamut Pasta	½ cup cooked, 70g	45-50	10	21g
Mexican Lasagna	½ cup, 120g	50	7.5	17.5g

GRAINS, CEREALS & PASTA	SERVING SIZE	GI	GL	NET CARB
Millet Porridge	½ cup cooked, 100g	50-70	7	12g
Oat Bran	½ cup, 110g	55-60	5.5	12g
Oatmeal	½ cup cooked, 117g	55-65	8.5	13.5g
Oatmeal	½ cup, 117g	55-60	7	15g
Pesto Lasagna	½ cup, 120g	50	5	15g
Polenta	½ cup cooked, 64g	70-85	9	12g
Popcorn	3 cups popped, 24g	55-65	7	15g
Quinoa	½ cup cooked, 185g	53	5	17g
Quinoa Porridge	½ cup cooked, 93g	50-65	6.5	11.5g
Rice Bran	½ cup, 58g	20-25	3	9g
Rye	1 slice of bread, 32g	57-62	10	14g
Rye Grain	½ cup cooked, 87g	45-50	7	15g
Seafood Lasagna	½ cup, 240g	50	5	12.5g
Semolina Porridge	½ cup cooked, 83g	50-65	6.5	11g
Shirataki Spaghetti	1 cup, 160g	0	0	0g
Soba	½ cup cooked, 57g	45	9.5	21g
Sorghum	½ cup cooked, 96g	65	9.5	14.5g
Spelt Pasta	½ cup cooked, 70g	44-49	9.5	20.5g
Spinach Lasagna	½ cup, 120g	50	6	15g
Steel-Cut Oats	½ cup cooked, 120g	55	7.5	13.5g
Teff	½ cup, 126g	45-50	8.5	21g
Teff Porridge	½ cup cooked, 120g	60-75	9	14.5g
Traditional Lasagna	½ cup, 120g	50	7	18g
Triticale	½ cup cooked, 182g	45-50	9.5	20g
Vegetarian Lasagna	½ cup, 120g	50	5	12.5g
Vermicelli Made from Soybeans	½ cup cooked, 150g	20-25	2.5	6g
Wheat Bran Crude	1 cup, 58g	40-45	7	20g
Wheat Germ Crude	½ cup, 58g	40-45	7.5	19.5g

GRAINS, CEREALS & PASTA	SERVING SIZE	GI	GL	NET CARB
Wheat Sprouted	½ cup, 55g	45-50	8.5	15.5g
Wild Barley	½ cup cooked, 87g	28-35	5	18g
Wild Rice	½ cup cooked, 82g	45-55	8	16g
MEDIUM GLYCEMIC LOAD FOODS *(consider reducing the serving size to stay below 15 grams of net carbs)*				
Angel Hair Spaghetti	½ cup cooked, 70g	45	11	25g
Arborio Rice	½ cup cooked, 100g	70	17.5	25g
Basmati Rice	½ cup cooked, 80g	58	12	19g
Brown Basmati Rice	½ cup cooked, 97g	55	10.5	19g
Brown Jasmine Rice	½ cup cooked, 97g	55	11.5	17g
Brown Rice	½ cup cooked, 98g	55	10.5	19g
Brown Rice Noodles	½ cup cooked, 90g	65	13	20g
Bucatini	½ cup cooked, 70g	55	12.2	25g
Capellini	½ cup cooked, 70g	55	13.75	25g
Carnaroli Rice	½ cup cooked, 100g	70	17.5	25g
Carrot Spaghetti	½ cup cooked, 70g	45	11	24.5g
Chow Mein Noodles	½ cup cooked, 70g	45	11	23g
Congee	½ cup cooked, 125g	75	15	22.5g
Corn Grain White	½ cup boiled, 164g	55-60	13.5	22.5g
Corn Grain Yellow	1 cup boiled, 164g	55-60	13.5	22.5g
Cornmeal	¼ cup dry, 30g	69	15	20g
Couscous	½ cup cooked, 79g	65	11	18g
Egg Noodles	½ cup cooked, 70g	40	10	25g
Farro	½ cup cooked, 84g	40	9	22g
Mushroom Lasagna	½ cup, 120g	50	6.5	16.5g
Rice Noodles	½ cup cooked, 85g	55	11	20g
Texmati Rice	½ cup cooked, 80g	60	11	20g

FISH, SEAFOOD, AND FISH PRODUCTS

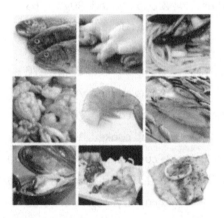

Fish, seafood, and fish products are a key part of many diets and offer unique benefits for those pursuing Reverse Type 2 Diabetes Diet. When considering their inclusion, one must assess their glycemic load (GL), nutritional content, and compatibility with Reverse Type 2 Diabetes Diet. By comprehending the benefits and potential drawbacks of fish, seafood, and fish products, individuals can make informed dietary decisions that support diabetes management and overall health.

Benefits of Fish and Seafood:

- **Rich in Omega-3 Fatty Acids**: Some fish, especially fatty ones like salmon, mackerel, and sardines, are excellent omega-3 fatty acids sources, which are known for their heart health benefits.
- **High-Quality Protein:** Fish and seafood are excellent sources of high-quality protein, which can help to maintain muscle mass and promote feelings of fullness.
- **Low Glycemic Load:** Fish and seafood have a low GL, meaning they have minimal impact on blood sugar levels.
- **Key Nutrients:** Fish and seafood provide essential nutrients like protein, omega-3 fatty acids, vitamin D, and Vitamin E, which can contribute to maintaining stable blood sugar and insulin levels.

Potential Drawbacks of Fish and Seafood:

- **Mercury Levels:** Some fish, particularly larger predatory fish (e.g., swordfish, tuna), can contain high levels of mercury.
- **Cooking Methods:** Some cooking methods, such as deep frying, can add unhealthy fats and increase the GL of fish and seafood. Breading or flouring can also raise the glycemic load of these foods.
- **Fish By-Products:** Highly processed fish products, like fish nuggets, sticks, or surimi, often contain high levels of unhealthy additives and sodium.

Incorporating Fish and Seafood into Reverse Type 2 Diabetes Diet:

When incorporating fish and seafood into your diet, consider the following tips:

- **Opt for Low-Mercury Fish:** Low-mercury fish like salmon, sardines, and trout are excellent choices.

- **Healthy Cooking Methods:** Opt for healthier cooking methods such as grilling, baking, broiling, or steaming to avoid adding excessive fats. Avoid frying or cooking methods that use a lot of added fats.

* * *

The following section of this chapter presents comprehensive tables of foods that are fully compliant with Reverse Type 2 Diabetes Diet. Each entry is accompanied by crucial information such as serving size, Glycemic Index (GI), Glycemic Load (GL), and Net Carbohydrates, enabling the reader to make informed decisions about portion sizes and meal planning.

However, it's important to note that not all compliant foods are equal. Some foods, while fitting within the parameters of the Reverse Type 2 Diabetes Diet, are more beneficial than others. For instance, foods that are minimally processed, lower in sodium, and rich in healthy fats are preferable. For these food items, even though GI, GL, and net carb data might not be the sole determinants of their suitability, their overall nutritional profile makes them excellent choices.

This distinction between different compliant foods enhances clarity and helps readers understand why certain foods are more desirable within the framework of the Reverse Type 2 Diabetes Diet. It also guides readers towards making healthier choices that align with the principles of this dietary approach and contribute to sustainable and effective diabetes management.

FISH, SEAFOODS & PRODUCTS

FISH, SEAFOODS & PRODUCTS	SERVING SIZE	GI	GL	NET CARB
Albacore Tuna	3 oz (85g)	0	0	0g
Amberjack	3 oz (85g)	0	0	0g
Anchovies	3 oz (85g)	0	0	0g
Barramundi	3 oz (85g)	0	0	0g
Black Drum	3 oz (85g)	0	0	0g
Black Sea Bass	3 oz (85g)	0	0	0g
Blackfin Tuna	3 oz (85g)	0	0	0g
Bluefin Tuna	3 oz (85g)	0	0	0g
Bluefish	3 oz (85g)	0	0	0g
Cajun Spiced Salmon Salad, low-carb dressing	7oz (200g)	45	4	9g
Canned Mackerel (in water)	3 oz (85g)	0	0	0g
Canned Salmon (in water)	3 oz (85g)	0	0	0g
Canned Sardines (in water)	3 oz (85g)	0	0	0g
Canned Trout (in water)	3 oz (85g)	0	0	0g
Canned Tuna (in water)	3 oz (85g)	0	0	1g
Catfish	3 oz (85g)	0	0	0g
Caviar	1 tbsp (16g)	0	0	0g
Ceviche Salad	7oz (200g)	40	2	6g
Clams	3 oz (85g)	0	0	2g
Cobia	3 oz (85g)	0	0	0g
Cod	3 oz (85g)	0	0	0g
Crab	3 oz (85g)	0	0	0g

FISH, SEAFOODS & PRODUCTS	SERVING SIZE	GI	GL	NET CARB
Crab and Avocado Salad, low-carb dressing	7oz (200g)	35	2	5g
Crab and Mango Salad, low-carb dressing	7oz (200g)	35	2	6g
Crab and Watermelon Salad, low-carb dressing	7oz (200g)	40	2	6g
Crab Louie Salad, low-carb dressing	8oz (250g)	35	2	7g
Crab Quinoa Salad, low-carb dressing	7oz (200g)	35	2	6g
Crayfish	3 oz (85g)	0	0	0g
Croaker	3 oz (85g)	0	0	0g
Drum	3 oz (85g)	0	0	0g
Fish and Chips	1 serving (350g)	55	50	90g
Fish and Vegetable Skewers	1 skewer (100g)	55	8	15g
Fish Ball	1 ball (25g)	55	2	3g
Fish Burger	1 patty (85g)	55	12	22g
Fish Fillet	1 fillet (85g)	55	12	22g
Fish Patty Sandwich	1 sandwich (200g)	55	17	30g
Fish Sandwich	1 sandwich (200g)	55	22	40g
Fish Taco	1 taco (150g)	55	14	26g
Fish Tacos	1 taco (150g)	55	14	26g
Fish Wrap	1 wrap (200g)	55	22	40g
Flounder	3 oz (85g)	0	0	0g
Greek Salmon Salad, low-carb dressing	7oz (200g)	40	3	8g
Grilled Shrimp and Quinoa Salad	7oz (200g)	40	3	8g
Grouper	3 oz (85g)	0	0	0g

FISH, SEAFOODS & PRODUCTS	SERVING SIZE	GI	GL	NET CARB
Haddock	3 oz (85g)	0	0	0g
Halibut	3 oz (85g)	0	0	0g
Herring	3 oz (85g)	0	0	0g
King Mackerel	3 oz (85g)	0	0	0g
Lake Trout	3 oz (85g)	0	0	0g
Lingcod	3 oz (85g)	0	0	0g
Lobster	3 oz (85g)	0	0	0g
Lobster Cobb Salad	8oz (250g)	40	3	8g
Lobster Mango Salad	7oz (200g)	35	2	7g
Mackerel	3 oz (85g)	0	0	0g
Marlin	3 oz (85g)	0	0	0g
Mediterranean Octopus Salad, low-carb dressing	7oz (200g)	40	2	6g
Monkfish	3 oz (85g)	0	0	0g
Mussels	3 oz (85g)	0	0	3g
Octopus	3 oz (85g)	0	0	0g
Oysters	3 oz (85g)	0	0	3g
Parrotfish	3 oz (85g)	0	0	0g
Pink Snapper	3 oz (85g)	0	0	0g
Pollock	3 oz (85g)	0	0	0g
Pompano	3 oz (85g)	0	0	0g
Rainbow Trout	3 oz (85g)	0	0	0g
Red Drum	3 oz (85g)	0	0	0g
Red Snapper	3 oz (85g)	0	0	0g
Redfish	3 oz (85g)	0	0	0g
Rockfish	3 oz (85g)	0	0	0g
Sablefish	3 oz (85g)	0	0	0g
Salmon	3 oz (85g)	0	0	0g

FISH, SEAFOODS & PRODUCTS	SERVING SIZE	GI	GL	NET CARB
Salmon Caesar Salad, low-carb dressing	7oz (200g)	45	4	8g
Salmon Spinach Salad, low-carb dressing	7oz (200g)	40	3	7g
Sardines	3 oz (85g)	0	0	0g
Scallop Salad, low-carb dressing	7oz (200g)	40	2	5g
Scallops	3 oz (85g)	0	0	2g
Seared Ahi Tuna Salad	7oz (200g)	40	3	7g
Seared Scallop and Grapefruit Salad, low-carb dressing	7oz (200g)	35	2	5g
Seared Scallops and Asparagus Salad, low-carb dressing	7oz (200g)	35	2	5g
Seared Swordfish Salad	7oz (200g)	40	3	7g
Sheepshead	3 oz (85g)	0	0	0g
Shrimp	3 oz (85g)	0	0	0g
Shrimp Avocado Salad, low-carb dressing	7oz (200g)	35	2	6g
Shrimp Cobb Salad	7oz (200g)	40	3	8g
Skate	3 oz (85g)	0	0	0g
Spicy Tuna Salad, low-carb dressing	7oz (200g)	45	3	7g
Squid	3 oz (85g)	0	0	0g
Striped Bass	3 oz (85g)	0	0	0g
Striped Marlin	3 oz (85g)	0	0	0g
Surimi	3 oz (85g)	25	1	5g
Swordfish	3 oz (85g)	0	0	0g
Tautog	3 oz (85g)	0	0	0g
Thai Shrimp Salad, low-carb dressing	7oz (200g)	35	2	7g

FISH, SEAFOODS & PRODUCTS	SERVING SIZE	GI	GL	NET CARB
Thai Squid Salad, low-carb dressing	7oz (200g)	40	2	6g
Tilapia	3 oz (85g)	0	0	0g
Tilefish	3 oz (85g)	0	0	0g
Triggerfish	3 oz (85g)	0	0	0g
Trout	3 oz (85g)	0	0	0g
Tuna	3 oz (85g)	0	0	0g
Tuna and White Bean Salad, low-carb dressing	7oz (200g)	35	2	6g
Tuna Nicoise Salad, low-carb dressing	8oz (250g)	50	5	10g
Tuna Pasta Salad, low-carb dressing	7oz (200g)	45	4	9g
Wahoo	3 oz (85g)	0	0	0g
White Bass	3 oz (85g)	0	0	0g
White Perch	3 oz (85g)	0	0	0g
Whitefish	3 oz (85g)	0	0	0g
Wrasse	3 oz (85g)	0	0	0g
Yellowfin Tuna	3 oz (85g)	0	0	0g
Yellowtail	3 oz (85g)	0	0	0g
Yellowtail Amberjack	3 oz (85g)	0	0	0g

FRUITS AND FRUITS PRODUCTS

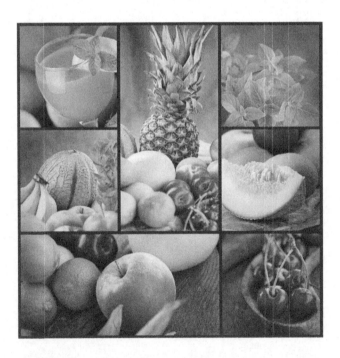

Fruits and their by-products form a fundamental part of many diets globally, and they're also essential for individuals pursuing Reverse Type 2 Diabetes Diet. Evaluating their glycemic load (GL), nutritional content, and suitability for a Reverse Type 2 Diabetes Diet is crucial. Knowing the benefits and potential drawbacks of fruits and fruit products can help individuals make educated dietary choices that support diabetes management and overall health.

Benefits of Fruits and Fruit Products:

- **Rich in Nutrients:** Fruits are packed with essential nutrients such as vitamins, minerals, trace minerals, and dietary fiber, all of which contribute to overall health and well-being.
- **Low in Fat and Calories:** Most fruits are low in fat and calories, making them a good choice for weight management.
- **High in Fiber:** Fruits are a great source of dietary fiber, which reduces the absorption of sugar into the bloodstream and prevents abrupt increases in blood glucose and insulin levels.

Potential Drawbacks of Fruits and Fruit Products:

- **Sugar Content:** Some fruits and fruit products, mainly processed ones, can contain high amounts of natural and added sugars, leading to potential spikes in blood glucose levels.
- **Processed Fruit Products:** Processed fruit products, like canned fruits, fruit juices, and dried fruits, can have added sugars and lower fiber content, making them less ideal for those managing diabetes.

Incorporating Fruits and Fruit Products into your eating plan:

- **Choose Whole Fruits:** Whole fruits are generally a better choice than processed fruit products, as they contain more fiber and fewer added sugars.
- **Monitor Portion Sizes:** Although fruits are healthy, they still contain carbohydrates and sugars, so portion control is essential.

- **Read Labels Diligently:** Pay careful attention to labels when purchasing fruit products. Look for products without added sugars and with high fiber content.

* * *

The following section of this chapter presents comprehensive tables of foods that are fully compliant with Reverse Type 2 Diabetes Diet. Each entry is accompanied by crucial information such as serving size, Glycemic Index (GI), Glycemic Load (GL), and Net Carbohydrates, enabling the reader to make informed decisions about portion sizes and meal planning.

However, it's important to note that not all compliant foods are equal. Some foods, while fitting within the parameters of the Reverse Type 2 Diabetes Diet, are more beneficial than others. For instance, foods that are minimally processed, lower in sodium, and rich in healthy fats are preferable. For these food items, even though GI, GL, and net carb data might not be the sole determinants of their suitability, their overall nutritional profile makes them excellent choices.

This distinction between different compliant foods enhances clarity and helps readers understand why certain foods are more desirable within the framework of the Reverse Type 2 Diabetes Diet. It also guides readers towards making healthier choices that align with the principles of this dietary approach and contribute to sustainable and effective diabetes management.

FRUITS & FRUIT PRODUCTS

FRUITS & FRUIT PRODUCTS	SERVING SIZE	GI	GL	NET CARB
LOW GLYCEMIC LOAD FOOD (Consider reducing the serving size to stay below 15 grams of net carbs)				
Acai	½ cup (100g) pulp	40	2	5g
Abiyuch	½ cup (64g)	45	7.2	16g
Acerola	1 cup (98g)	25	2	8g
Acerola Juice	½ cup (120ml)	30-40	2.4	6g
Ackee	½ cup (100g)	50	4	8g
African Cherry Orange	1 fruit (40g)	40	2	4g
African Cucumber	½ cup (60g)	40	2	4g
Apple	1 medium (182g)	36	5	21g
Apple Baked Unsweetened	1 cup (125g)	35-40	8	23g
Apple Butter	1 tbsp (20g)	40-45	6	10g
Apple Chips	1 cup (30g)	45-50	10	22g
Apple Juice	½ cup (120ml)	45	6.3	14g
Apple Juice Concentrate	¼ cup (60g)	40	12	15g
Apple Pickled	½ cup (75g)	30-35	4	12g
Applesauce, Canned Light Syrup Drained	¼ cup (61g)	40	5	12.5g
Apricot	1 fruit (35g)	34	2	4g
Apricot Jam	1 tbsp (20g)	50-55	8	13g
Apricot Juice Concentrate	¼ cup (60g)	40	6	12g
Apricot Plum	1 fruit (50g)	34	2	7g
Apricots, Canned Light Syrup Drained	½ cup (122g)	40-45	7	14g
Asian Pears	1 medium (166g)	30-35	6	17g

FRUITS & FRUIT PRODUCTS	SERVING SIZE	GI	GL	NET CARB
Avocado	½ medium (100g)	15	0.3	2g
Babaco	½ cup (75g)	30	2	5g
Banana Passionfruit	1 fruit (20g)	35	1	3g
Barbados Cherry	½ cup (75g)	30	2	6g
Bartlett Pears	1 medium (166g)	30-35	6	20g
Beet Juice	½ cup (120ml)	64	5	11g
Black Sapote	½ cup (50g)	35	3	9g
Blackberries	1 cup (144g)	25-30	3	10g
Blackberries, Canned Light Syrup Drained	½ cup (122g)	25	3	8g
Blackberry	½ cup (72g)	25	2	7g
Blackberry Jam	1 tbsp (20g)	50-55	8	13g
Blackcurrant Juice Concentrate	¼ cup (60g)	20	0	0g
Blueberries	1 cup (148g)	40-45	6	17g
Blueberries Canned Light Syrup Drained	1 cup (230g)	40-45	10	23g
Blueberries, Canned Light Syrup Drained	½ cup (122g)	40	7	15g
Blueberry	½ cup (75g)	40	4	10g
Blueberry Jam	1 tbsp (20g)	50-55	8	13g
Blueberry Juice	½ cup (120ml)	40	5.8	14g
Blueberry Juice Concentrate	¼ cup (60g)	55	6.3	12g
Boysenberries	1 cup (144g)	25-30	4	12g
Boysenberry	½ cup (75g)	30	3	8g
Breadfruit	½ cup (60g)	60	6	12g
California Avocados	½ avocado (100g)	15-20	1	3g
California Grapefruit	1 medium (154g)	25-30	4	13g

FRUITS & FRUIT PRODUCTS	SERVING SIZE	GI	GL	NET CARB
California Valencia Oranges	1 medium (131g)	40-45	6	14g
Cantaloupe	½ cup (89g)	60	4	7g
Cape Gooseberry	½ cup (50g)	40	3	7g
Carambola (starfruit)	1 fruit (92g)	30	2	6g
Carissa	1 cup (132g)	35-40	7	18g
Carrot Juice	½ cup (120ml)	43	4.1	9.5g
Casaba Melon	1 cup (160g)	30-35	4	11g
Cempedak	½ cup (75g)	40	4	10g
Cherimoya	½ fruit (85g)	35	3	9g
Cherries, Canned Light Syrup Drained	½ cup (122g)	55-60	9	18g
Cherry	½ cup (76g)	22	3	10g
Cherry Juice	½ cup (120ml)	50	7	14g
Cherry Preserves	1 tbsp (20g)	50-55	8	13g
Chokeberry	½ cup (60g)	35	2	6g
Clementine	1 fruit (74g)	35	3	9g
Cloudberry	½ cup (60g)	25	2	5g
Coconut	½ cup (40g) shredded	45	2	5g
Cornelian Cherry	½ cup (75g)	30	2	6g
Cranberry	½ cup (50g)	45	3	6g
Cranberry Juice	½ cup (120ml)	52	7.5	15g
Cranberry Juice Concentrate	¼ cup (60g)	50	5	10g
Cranberry Sauce	1 tbsp (20g)	50-55	8	13g
Currant	½ cup (56g)	25	2	8g
Damson	½ cup (75g)	30	3	8g
Date	¼ cup (30g)	42	10	24g
Date Plum	1 fruit (25g)	35	2	5g

FRUITS & FRUIT PRODUCTS	SERVING SIZE	GI	GL	NET CARB
Desert Lime	1 fruit (30g)	30	1	3g
Dragonfruit	½ fruit (100g)	30	2	6g
Dried Apple	¼ cup (28g)	44	10	16g
Dried Coconut	¼ cup (20g)	40	3	7g
Dried Dragon Fruit	¼ cup (28g)	55	9	15g
Dried Goji Berries	¼ cup (28g)	29	7	14g
Dried Guava	¼ cup (30g)	45	10	18g
Dried Peach	¼ cup (36g)	35	10	20g
Dried Raspberries	¼ cup (30g)	40	8	16g
Dried Strawberries	¼ cup (30g)	50	10	18g
Durian	½ cup (100g)	45	6	13g
Elderberry	½ cup (50g)	25	2	6g
Feijoa	1 fruit (50g)	35	2	6g
Fig	1 medium (50g)	60	8	14g
Fig Preserves	1 tbsp (20g)	50-55	8	13g
Finger Lime	1 fruit (10g)	30	0	1g
Fruit cocktail, Canned Light Syrup Drained	½ cup (122g)	55	8	16g
Gac Fruit	¼ cup (25g) pulp	30	1	2g
Galia Melon	½ cup (90g)	65	4	6g
Genip	1 fruit (20g)	35	1	3g
Goji Berries Dried	¼ cup (28g)	35-40	5	12g
Golden Delicious Apples	1 medium (174g)	35-40	6	17g
Goldenberry	½ cup (50g)	35	3	6g
Gooseberry	½ cup (75g)	25	2	8g
Granny Smith Apples	1 medium (170g)	30-35	5	14g
Grape	½ cup (75g)	46	5	13g
Grape Jelly	1 tbsp (20g)	50-55	8	13g
Grapefruit	1 medium (154g)	25-30	4	13g

FRUITS & FRUIT PRODUCTS	SERVING SIZE	GI	GL	NET CARB
Grapefruit Juice	½ cup (120ml)	48	5	11g
Grapefruit segments, Canned Light Syrup Drained	½ cup (122g)	25	3	10g
Grapes	½ cup (76g)	45-50	4	9g
Graviola (Soursop)	½ cup (100g) pulp	40	4	10g
Greengage	1 fruit (20g)	30	1	3g
Groundcherries	1 cup (140g)	35-40	7	20g
Guanabana	½ cup (100g) pulp	40	4	10g
Guava	1 medium (55g)	20	1	4g
Guava Juice	½ cup (120ml)	33	3.3	10g
Guava, Canned Light Syrup Drained	½ cup (122g)	35-50	5	10g
Hala Fruit	¼ cup (25g) pulp	35	1	2g
Honeydew Melon	½ cup (85g)	60	4	8g
Huckleberry	½ cup (75g)	25	2	6g
Imbe	1 fruit (20g)	40	1	2g
Jabuticaba	½ cup (50g)	35	3	6g
Jackfruit	½ cup (100g)	50	8	16g
Jambul	½ cup (75g)	30	2	5g
Japanese Plum	1 fruit (40g)	40	2	4g
Jujube	1 fruit (15g)	50	3	6g
Jumbo Olives	¼ cup (40g)	15-Oct	0	1g
Kaffir Lime	1 fruit (30g)	30	1	2g
Kei Apple	1 fruit (20g)	35	1	3g
Kitembilla	½ cup (50g)	30	2	5g
Kiwano (Horned Melon)	½ fruit (100g)	35	2	7g
Kiwi	1 fruit (69g)	50	5	9g

FRUITS & FRUIT PRODUCTS	SERVING SIZE	GI	GL	NET CARB
Kumquat	5 fruits (50g)	30	3	6g
Langsat	½ cup (75g)	40	3	8g
Lemon	1 fruit (58g)	20	1	3g
Lemon Curd	1 tbsp (20g)	50-55	8	13g
Lemon Juice	½ cup (120ml)	20	2	10.5g
Lemon Juice Concentrate	1 tbsp (15g)	20	0.2	1g
Lime	1 fruit (44g)	20	1	3g
Lime Juice Concentrate	1 tbsp (15g)	20	0.2	1g
Limequat	1 fruit (20g)	30	1	2g
Loganberries	1 cup (180g)	25-30	3	9g
Longan	½ cup (50g)	50	5	10g
Loquat	½ cup (75g)	35	2	5g
Lychee	½ cup (75g)	50	6	12g
Mandarin Orange	1 fruit (88g)	40	4	9g
Mandarin oranges, Canned Light Syrup Drained	½ cup (122g)	45	6	13g
Mango	½ cup (83g)	55	8	15g
Mango Jam	1 tbsp (20g)	50-55	8	13g
Mango Juice	½ cup (120ml)	41	6.2	15g
Mango Pickled	¼ cup (60g)	40-45	6	12g
Mango, Canned Light Syrup Drained	½ cup (122g)	40-50	8	16g
Mangosteen	1 fruit (75g)	45	3	6g
Marula	1 fruit (10g)	30	1	1g
Medlar	1 fruit (20g)	35	1	3g
Melon	1 cup (177g)	65	5	12g
Miracle Fruit	1 fruit (5g)	30	0	1g
Mixed Berry Jam	1 tbsp (20g)	50-55	8	13g

FRUITS & FRUIT PRODUCTS	SERVING SIZE	GI	GL	NET CARB
Mulberry	½ cup (70g)	25	3	6g
Nagami Kumquat	5 fruits (50g)	30	3	6g
Nance	1 cup (120g)	40-45	10	20g
Navel Oranges	1 medium (154g)	35-40	6	15g
Nectarine	1 medium (142g)	40	4	11g
Nectarines	1 medium (142g)	35-40	6	15g
Oheloberries	1 cup (140g)	30-35	5	11g
Okra Pickled	1 cup (160g)	15-20	1	3g
Olive	5 large (25g)	15	0	1g
Orange	1 medium (131g)	40	4	12g
Orange Juice	½ cup (120ml)	50	6.5	13g
Orange Marmalade	1 tbsp (20g)	50-55	8	13g
Papaya	1 cup (145g)	60	6	11g
Papaya, Canned Light Syrup Drained	½ cup (122g)	55-60	7	14g
Passion Fruit	1 fruit (18g)	30	1	2g
Passionfruit Juice	½ cup (120ml)	30	2.1	7g
Passionfruit Juice Concentrate	¼ cup (60g)	35	3	8.7g
Pawpaw	1 cup (140g)	60	6	11g
Peach	1 medium (150g)	40	4	10g
Peach Juice	½ cup (120ml)	42	6	14g
Peach Juice Concentrate	¼ cup (60g)	40	6	12g
Peach Pickled	½ cup (130g)	40-45	8	16g
Peach Preserves	1 tbsp (20g)	50-55	8	13g
Peaches, Canned Light Syrup Drained	½ cup (122g)	40-45	8	16g
Pear	1 medium (178g)	38	5	21g
Pear Juice	½ cup (120ml)	44	5.5	14g

FRUITS & FRUIT PRODUCTS	SERVING SIZE	GI	GL	NET CARB
Pears Canned Extra Light Syrup	½ cup (122g)	40-45	5.5	11g
Pears, Canned Light Syrup Drained	½ cup (122g)	43	7	15g
Peppers Pickled	1 cup (150g)	15-20	1	3g
Persimmon	1 fruit (25g)	50	3	6g
Pineapple	½ cup (82g)	59	7	10g
Pineapple Juice	½ cup (120ml)	46	6.5	14g
Pineapple Preserves	1 tbsp (20g)	50-55	8	13g
Pineapple, Canned Extra Light Syrup	½ cup (122g)	50-55	7.5	15g
Pitanga	1 cup (140g)	35-40	7	14g
Plum	1 fruit (66g)	40	2	6g
Plum Jam	1 tbsp (20g)	50-55	8	13g
Plum Pickled	1 cup (150g)	30-35	6	12g
Plums Canned Extra Purple Light Syrup	½ cup (122g)	40-45	6.7	15g
Plums, Canned Light Syrup Drained	½ cup (122g)	40	6	12g
Pomegranate	½ cup (87g)	53	6	12g
Pomegranate Juice	½ cup (120ml)	53	9	17g
Pomegranate Juice Concentrate	¼ cup (60g)	35	8	12g
Pomelo	½ fruit (154g)	30	3	9g
Prickly Pear	1 fruit (103g)	35	2	5g
Prunes	¼ cup (40g)	29	10	18g
Pummelo	1 cup sections (190g)	30-35	4	8g
Purple Passion Fruit Juice	½ cup (120ml)	30-35	5	10g
Quince	1 fruit (92g)	34	2	6g
Quince Jelly	1 tbsp (20g)	50-55	8	13g

FRUITS & FRUIT PRODUCTS	SERVING SIZE	GI	GL	NET CARB
Raspberries, Canned Light Syrup Drained	½ cup (122g)	32	3	9g
Raspberry	½ cup (62g)	32	1	3g
Raspberry Jam	1 tbsp (20g)	50-55	8	13g
Raspberry Juice Concentrate	¼ cup (60g)	40	5	10g
Red Banana	1 medium (100g)	45	7	18g
Red Currant Jelly	1 tbsp (20g)	50-55	8	13g
Redcurrant	½ cup (56g)	25	2	5g
Rhubarb	1 cup (122g)	15	1	3g
Rose Apple	1 fruit (45g)	30	1	3g
Santa Claus Melon	1 cup (177g)	60	6	13g
Sapodilla	1 fruit (150g)	45	6	14g
Soursop	1 cup (225g)	45	6	15g
Star Apple	1 fruit (138g)	35	3	6g
Star Fruit	1 fruit (91g)	25	1	4g
Strawberries, Canned Light Syrup Drained	½ cup (122g)	40	4	10g
Strawberry	½ cup (72g)	32	1	4g
Strawberry Jam	1 tbsp (20g)	50-55	8	13g
Strawberry Juice Concentrate	¼ cup (60g)	40	5	10g
Sweet Granadilla	1 fruit (140g)	40	3	10g
Tahitian Pomelo	½ fruit (154g)	40	4	10g
Tamarind	1 oz (28g)	40	3	6g
Tangelo	1 fruit (109g)	42	4	10g
Tangerine	1 fruit (84g)	40	3	9g
Tomato Juice	1 cup (240ml)	38	3.8	10g
Tsukemono Japanese Pickles	1 cup (150g)	15-20	2	4g

FRUITS & FRUIT PRODUCTS	SERVING SIZE	GI	GL	NET CARB
Turnip Pickled	1 cup (150g)	15-20	1	3g
Ugli Fruit	½ fruit (120g)	40	4	10g
Ugni Fruit	¼ cup (30g)	30	2	4g
Vanilla Bean	1 bean (6g)	50	1	1g
Velvet Apple	1 fruit (166g)	35	3	9g
Wampi	¼ cup (28g)	30	1	3g
Watermelon	1 cup (152g)	72	5	11g
Watermelon Juice	½ cup (120ml)	72	7.2	9g
White Currant	½ cup (56g)	25	2	5g
White Sapote	1 fruit (170g)	30	2	6g
Yellow Passion Fruit	1 fruit (18g)	30	1	2g
Yellow Watermelon	1 cup (152g)	72	5	11g
Yuzu	1 fruit (77g)	30	1	2g
Zante Currant	¼ cup (40g)	60	10	17g
Ziziphus Fruit	1 fruit (10g)	35	1	3g
Zombie Fruit (a type of passion fruit)	1 fruit (18g)	30	1	2g
Zucchini Squash	1 cup (124g)	15	1	3g
Zwetschge (a type of plum)	1 fruit (66g)	40	2	5g
MEDIUM GLYCEMIC LOAD FOOD *(Consider reducing the serving size to stay below 15 grams of net carbs)*				
Ambrosia	½ cup (120g)	54	10.8	20g
Banana	1 extra small (105g)	51-65	15.6	24g
Banana Baked	1 extra small (105g)	60-60	19.3	28g
Dates	¼cup (40g)	42	18	28g
Dried Apricots, Unsweetened	¼ cup (32g)	32	12	18g

FRUITS & FRUIT PRODUCTS	SERVING SIZE	GI	GL	NET CARB
Dried Banana, Unsweetened	¼cup (30g)	54	14	22g
Dried Blueberries, Unsweetened	¼ cup (40g)	53	14	26g
Dried Cherries, Unsweetened	¼ cup (40g)	54	16	30g
Dried Cranberries, Unsweetened	¼ cup (40g)	64	18	28g
Dried Currants, Unsweetened	¼ cup (40g)	56	17	30g
Dried Custard Apple, Unsweetened	¼ cup (30g)	48	13	22g
Dried Kiwi, Unsweetened	¼ cup (30g)	54	11	19g
Dried Longan, Unsweetened	¼ cup (32g)	55	15	28g
Dried Lychee, Unsweetened	¼ cup (30g)	52	13	22g
Dried Mango, Unsweetened	¼ cup (30g)	55	12	22g
Dried Papaya, Unsweetened	¼ cup (30g)	60	15	25g
Dried Pear, Unsweetened	¼ cup (40g)	43	12	24g
Dried Persimmon, Unsweetened	¼ cup (32g)	53	15	24g
Dried Pineapple, Unsweetened	¼ cup (35g)	58	16	28g
Dried Sapodilla, Unsweetened	¼ cup (30g)	50	12	20g
Figs	¼ cup (40g)	61	15	24g
Golden Seedless Raisins	¼ cup (40g)	50-55	17	31g
Grape Juice Concentrate	¼ cup (60g)	70	12	15g
Guava Nectar Canned	1 cup (240g)	40-45	15	30g
Guava Sauce Cooked	1 cup (250g)	40-45	14	28g
Litchis	1 cup (190g)	50-55	14	25g

FRUITS & FRUIT PRODUCTS	SERVING SIZE	GI	GL	NET CARB
Mango Cooked	1 cup (165g)	45-50	15	30g
Plantain	1 cup, sliced (148g)	40	12	30g
Prune Puree	¼ cup (60g)	40-45	12	24g
Prune Whip	1/2 cup (125g)	40-45	14	28g

BEEF, VEAL, PORK, LAMB AND POULTRY

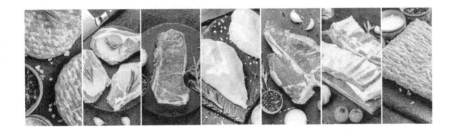

Meat products serve as an essential component of many diets, and they can fit well into Reverse Type 2 Diabetes Diet when chosen wisely and consumed in moderation. Understanding the glycemic load (GL), nutritional content, and the benefits and potential drawbacks of meat consumption can support individuals in making informed dietary decisions that align with diabetes management and overall health.

Benefits of Meat in a Diabetes Reversal Diet:

- **Nutrient Density:** Meat is a powerhouse of essential nutrients, including iron, zinc, and vitamins, especially B. These nutrients contribute to overall health and help prevent nutrient deficiencies often seen in individuals with diabetes.

- **Complete Protein Source:** Meat offers all nine essential amino acids that human bodies are incapable of producing on their own, making it a whole protein source. This is crucial for muscle growth, repair, and overall health. Given that individuals with type 2 diabetes may face challenges in maintaining sufficient protein intake, incorporating lean meats can be beneficial.

Potential Drawbacks of Meat:

- **Saturated Fats:** Certain meats, particularly fatty cuts, and processed variants, are high in saturated fats. Excessive intake of saturated fat promotes weight gain and increases the likelihood of heart disease, both detrimental to individuals managing type 2 diabetes.
- **Processed Meats:** Processed meats like sausages, bacon, and lunch meats often contain high amounts of sodium, nitrates, and additives that may negatively affect health. These meats are generally not recommended for Reverse Type 2 Diabetes Diet.

Guidelines for Incorporating Meat into Reverse Type 2 Diabetes Diet:

- **Choose Lean Meats:** Opt for lean meats such as lean cuts of red meat, skinless poultry, and fish. These choices contain less saturated fat and fewer calories, making them more compatible with a diet aimed at diabetes reversal and weight management.
- **Avoid Highly Processed Meats:** Highly processed meats are often high in sodium, additives, and unhealthy fats. These processed meats are not compliant with Reverse Type 2 Diabetes Diet.

- **Healthy Cooking Methods:** Employ healthy cooking methods such as grilling, baking, or steaming rather than frying to avoid adding unnecessary fats.
- **Serving Size and Nutritional Information:** Remember that the serving sizes and nutritional information provided in the tables in this chapter are tailored for meats compatible with Reverse Type 2 Diabetes Diet. These tables exclude high-sodium and excessively processed meats. The GI, GL, and net carb content per typical serving are calculated based on these healthy cooking methods and meat choices.

* * *

The following section of this chapter presents comprehensive tables of foods that are fully compliant with Reverse Type 2 Diabetes Diet. Each entry is accompanied by crucial information such as serving size, Glycemic Index (GI), Glycemic Load (GL), and Net Carbohydrates, enabling the reader to make informed decisions about portion sizes and meal planning.

However, it's important to note that not all compliant foods are equal. Some foods, while fitting within the parameters of the Reverse Type 2 Diabetes Diet, are more beneficial than others. For instance, foods that are minimally processed, lower in sodium, and rich in healthy fats are preferable. For these food items, even though GI, GL, and net carb data might not be the sole determinants of their suitability, their overall nutritional profile makes them excellent choices.

This distinction between different compliant foods enhances clarity and helps readers understand why certain foods are more desirable within the framework of the Reverse Type 2 Diabetes Diet. It also guides readers towards making healthier choices that align with the principles of this dietary approach and contribute to sustainable and effective diabetes management.

BEEF, PORK & POULTRY PRODUCTS

BEEF, PORK & POULTRY PRODUCTS	SERVING SIZE	GI	GL	NET CARB
Bacon, Uncured, low-sodium, no added sugar Grilled or Baked	3 slices, 35g	0	0	0g
Beef Brisket, Oven-Roasted	3 oz, 85g	0	0	0g
Beef Brisket, Slow-Cooked	3 oz, 85g	0	0	0g
Beef Burger, lean, Broiled	1 burger, 150g	0	0	0g
Beef Burger, lean, Grilled	1 burger, 150g	0	0	0g
Beef jerky, low-sodium	1 oz, 28g	0-5	0	3g
Beef Ribs, Slow-Cooked	3 ribs, 180g	0	0	0g
Beef Roast, Marinated and Oven-Roasted	4 oz, 113g	0	0	0g
Beef Roast, Oven-Roasted	4 oz, 113g	0	0	0g
Beef Roast, Slow-Cooked	4 oz, 113g	0	0	0g
Beef Roast, Slow-Cooked with Vegetables	4 oz, 113g	0	0	1g
Beef Sirloin, Broiled	4 oz, 113g	0	0	0g
Beef Sirloin, Grilled	4 oz, 113g	0	0	0g
Beef Sirloin, Marinated and Pan-Seared	4 oz, 113g	25-35	3	10g
Beef Sirloin, Pan-Seared	4 oz, 113g	0	0	0g
Beef Steak, Grilled	4 oz, 113g	0	0	0g
Beef Steak, Marinated and Grilled	4 oz, 113g	25-35	2	5g
Beef Steak, Marinated and Pan-Fried	4 oz, 113g	30-35	2	5g
Beef Steak, Oven-Baked	4 oz, 113g	0	0	0g
Beef Steak, Pan-Seared	4 oz, 113g	0	0	0g

BEEF, PORK & POULTRY PRODUCTS	SERVING SIZE	GI	GL	NET CARB
Beef Stew, Slow-Cooked	1 cup, 240g	0	0	0g
Beef Stew, with Carrots and Peas	1 cup, 240g	0	0	5g
Beef Stew, with Corn and Green Beans	1 cup, 240g	15-25	1	5g
Beef Stew, with Mushrooms	1 cup, 240g	15-25	1	5g
Beef sticks, low-sodium	1 oz, 28g	0	0	1g
Beef Stir-Fry, with Vegetables	1 cup, 200g	0	0	0g
Bison Burger, Grilled	1 patty	0	0	0g
Bison Steak, Grilled	3 oz	0	0	0g
Chicken Breast, Grilled	4 oz, 113g	0	0	0g
Chicken Breast, Marinated and Baked	4 oz, 113g	25-35	2	5g
Chicken Breast, Marinated and Grilled	4 oz, 113g	0-5	0	5g
Chicken Breast, Pan-Seared	4 oz, 113g	0	0	0g
Chicken Cutlet, Grilled	1 cutlet, 120g	20-30	1	5g
Chicken Drumstick, Baked	1 drumstick, 85g	0	0	0g
Chicken Drumstick, Roasted	1 drumstick, 85g	0	0	0g
Chicken Tender, Baked	4 tenders, 85g	40-55	3	5g
Chicken Thigh, Baked	1 thigh, 120g	0	0	0g
Chicken Thigh, Grilled	1 thigh, 120g	0	0	0g
Chuck roast, Grilled or Broiled	3 oz, 85g	0	0	0g
Cornish Game Hen, Roasted	1 hen	0	0	0g
Duck Breast, Pan-Seared	3 oz	0	0	0g
Duck Leg, Roasted	1 leg	0	0	0g
Elk Steak, Grilled	3 oz	0	0	0g

BEEF, PORK & POULTRY PRODUCTS	SERVING SIZE	GI	GL	NET CARB
Filet mignon, Grilled or Broiled	3 oz, 85g	0	0	0g
Flank steak, Grilled or Broiled	3 oz, 85g	0	0	0g
Goose, Roasted	3 oz	0	0	0g
Ground Beef, , Lean, low-sodium, homemade, Baked	3 oz, 85g	0	0	0g
Ground Beef, lean, low-sodium, Broiled	3 oz, 85g	0	0	0g
Ground Beef, lean, Lean, low-sodium, homemade, Grilled	3 oz, 85g	0	0	0g
Ground Beef, Lean, low-sodium, homemade, Pan-Fried	3 oz, 85g	0	0	0g
Ground Lamb, lean, low-sodium, Pan-Fried	3 oz	0	0	0g
Ground meat products, Lean, homemade Grilled or Broiled	3 oz, 85g	0	0	0g
Ground Pork, Pan-Fried	3 oz, 85g	40-55	2	5g
Ground Turkey, Baked	3 oz	0	0	0g
Ground Turkey, Pan-Fried	3 oz	0	0	0g
Lamb Chops, Grilled	3 oz	0	0	0g
Lamb Roast, Oven-Roasted	3 oz	0	0	0g
Lamb Shank, Braised	3 oz	0	0	0g
Ostrich Steak, Grilled	3 oz	0	0	0g
Pork Belly, Braised	3 oz, 85g	20-30	2	5g
Pork Belly, Roasted	3 oz, 85g	35-50	3	5g
Pork Loin Chop, Grilled	1 chop, 150g	20-30	3	5g
Pork Loin Roast, Oven-Roasted	3 oz, 85g	30-45	2	5g

BEEF, PORK & POULTRY PRODUCTS	SERVING SIZE	GI	GL	NET CARB
Pork Loin Roast, Slow-Cooked	4 oz, 113g	25-35	2	5g
Pork Loin, Oven-Baked	4 oz, 113g	30-45	1	5g
Pork Ribs, Slow-Cooked	3 ribs, 180g	25-35	3	5g
Pork Roast, Oven-Roasted	4 oz, 113g	35-50	3	5g
Pork Shoulder, Slow-Roasted	3 oz, 85g	50-65	3	5g
Pork Tenderloin, Marinated and Grilled	4 oz, 113g	25-35	2	5g
Quail, Grilled or Roasted	1 quail	0	0	0g
Rabbit, Braised or Grilled	3 oz	0	0	0g
Ribeye steak, Grilled or Broiled	3 oz, 85g	0	0	0g
Round steak, Grilled or Broiled	3 oz, 85g	0	0	0g
Sausage, Lean, Low-sodium, Grilled or Baked	3 oz, 85g	0	0	1g
Short ribs, Grilled or Broiled	3 oz, 85g	0	0	0g
Sirloin steak, Grilled or Broiled	3 oz, 85g	0	0	0g
Skirt steak, Grilled or Broiled	3 oz, 85g	0	0	0g
T-bone steak, Grilled or Broiled	3 oz, 85g	0	0	0g
Tri-tip, Grilled or Broiled	3 oz, 85g	0	0	0g
Turkey Breast, Roasted	3 oz	0	0	0g
Turkey Burger, lean, low-sodium, homemade, Grilled	1 patty	0	0	0g
Turkey Drumstick, Roasted	1 drumstick	0	0	0g
Turkey Tender, Baked	3 oz	0	0	0g
Turkey Thigh, Roasted	1 thigh	0	0	0g
Turkey Wing, Baked	1 wing	0	0	0g
Veal Roast, Oven-Roasted	3 oz	0	0	0g

BEEF, PORK & POULTRY PRODUCTS	SERVING SIZE	GI	GL	NET CARB
Veal Scallopini, Pan-Seared	3 oz	0	0	0g
Venison Steak, Grilled	3 oz	0	0	0g
Veal Roast, Oven-Roasted	3 oz	0	0	0g
Veal Scallopini, Pan-Seared	3 oz	0	0	0g

NUTS AND SEEDS

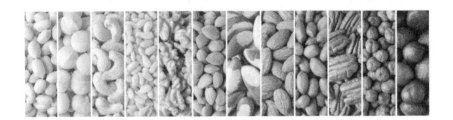

Nuts and seeds are a vital component of many diets, particularly for individuals following Reverse Type 2 Diabetes Diet. The potential benefits and drawbacks, along with strategies for their inclusion in such a diet, are essential to understand for successful dietary management of diabetes.

Benefits of Nuts and Seeds:

- **Nutrient-Rich:** Nuts and seeds are exceptionally nutrient-dense. They are packed with beneficial components such as fiber, protein, and healthy fats. Moreover, they provide a wealth of essential vitamins and minerals, including vitamin

E, zinc, calcium, and magnesium, all contributing to overall health and well-being.

- **Heart Health:** Nuts and seeds are rich in healthy fats (monounsaturated / polyunsaturated fats), which can help decrease levels of harmful LDL cholesterol and increase protective HDL cholesterol. This advantage translates to a reduced risk of heart disease, making these nutrient powerhouses an excellent choice for heart health.
- **Blood Sugar Control:** Due to their combined high fiber and protein content, nuts and seeds make digestion slow, resulting in a gradual release of glucose into the bloodstream, supporting blood sugar regulation. This is particularly advantageous for individuals with diabetes.
- **Antioxidant Content:** Many nuts and seeds are high in antioxidants, which combat oxidative stress in the body. Antioxidants can help prevent cellular damage and reduce inflammation, both of which are beneficial for managing diabetes.
- **Protein-Rich:** Nuts and seeds are an excellent source of plant-based protein. The protein content helps promote satiety, assisting in weight management, which is crucial for diabetes reversal.

Potential Drawbacks of Nuts and Seeds:

- **High in Calories:** Nuts and seeds are also high in calories due to their high nutrient density. While they offer numerous health benefits, it's important to moderate consumption to avoid potential weight gain.
- **Salted or Coated Varieties:** Many commercially available nuts and seeds are salted, sugar-coated, or processed with additional oils. These versions can add excessive sodium or sugars to your diet and should be avoided.

Incorporating Nuts and Seeds into Reverse Type 2 Diabetes Diet:

- **Choose Raw or Dry-Roasted:** Opt for raw or dry-roasted nuts and seeds. These forms are typically devoid of unhealthy added oils, sugars, or salts.
- **Monitor Portion Sizes:** Despite their health benefits, the high-calorie content of nuts and seeds means portion control is essential. A handful is typically an appropriate serving.
- **Ideal for Snacks:** Given their high protein and fiber content, nuts and seeds make for an ideal snack option. They can help manage hunger between meals, preventing overeating.
- **Include Nut and Seed Butter:** Nuts and seed butter (e.g., almond butter,tahini) can be a valuable addition to a Reverse Type 2 Diabetes Diet. These products offer the same benefits as whole nuts and seeds but in a versatile, spreadable form.
- **Versatile Addition:** Nuts and seeds can be added to a variety of dishes. Sprinkle them over salads, stir into oatmeal or yogurt, or use them to add crunch to a stir-fry.

* * *

The following section of this chapter presents comprehensive tables of foods that are fully compliant with Reverse Type 2 Diabetes Diet. Each entry is accompanied by crucial information such as serving size, Glycemic Index (GI), Glycemic Load (GL), and Net Carbohydrates, enabling the reader to make informed decisions about portion sizes and meal planning.

However, it's important to note that not all compliant foods are equal. Some foods, while fitting within the parameters of the Reverse Type 2 Diabetes Diet, are more beneficial than others. For instance, foods that are minimally processed, lower in sodium, and rich in healthy fats are preferable. For these food items, even though GI, GL, and net carb data might not be the sole determinants of their suitability, their overall nutritional profile makes them excellent choices.

This distinction between different compliant foods enhances clarity and helps readers understand why certain foods are more desirable within the framework of the Reverse Type 2 Diabetes Diet. It also guides readers towards making healthier choices that align with the principles of this dietary approach and contribute to sustainable and effective diabetes management.

NUTS & SEEDS

NUTS & SEEDS	SERVING SIZE	GI	GL	NET CARB
Almond Butter	2 tbsp (32g)	0	0	3g
Almonds	1 oz (28g)	0	0	2g
Boiled Chestnuts	1 oz (28g)	60	2	14g
Brazil Nut Butter	2 tbsp (32g)	15	1	2g
Brazil nuts	1 oz (28g)	15	0	1g
Butternuts	1 oz (28g)	15	0	2g
Cashew Butter	2 tbsp (32g)	25	3	6g
Cashews	1 oz (28g)	25	6	8g
Chestnuts	1 oz (28g)	60	2	14g
Chia Nut Butter	2 tbsp (32g)	1	1	2g
Chia nuts	1 oz (28g)	1	1	1g
Chia seeds	1 oz (28g)	1	1	2g
Coconut	1 oz (28g)	51	6	6g
Fennel seeds	1 oz (28g)	5	1	2g
Fenugreek seeds	1 oz (28g)	15	1	6g
Filbert (Hazelnut) Butter	2 tbsp (32g)	0	0	3g
Filberts (Hazelnuts)	1 oz (28g)	0	0	2g
Flaxseeds (Linseeds)	1 oz (28g)	55	1	0g
Hazelnut Butter	2 tbsp (32g)	15	1	3g
Hazelnuts	1 oz (28g)	15	0	2g
Hemp seeds	1 oz (28g)	0	0	1g
Macadamia Nut Butter	2 tbsp (32g)	15	1	3g
Macadamia nuts	1 oz (28g)	15	1	2g
Mustard seeds	1 oz (28g)	15	1	2g
Peanut Butter	2 tbsp (32g)	13	3	6g

NUTS & SEEDS	SERVING SIZE	GI	GL	NET CARB
Peanuts	1 oz (28g)	13	<1	3g
Pecan Butter	2 tbsp (32g)	0	0	2g
Pecans	1 oz (28g)	0	0	1g
Pine Nut Oil	1 tbsp (14g)	15	0	0g
Pine nuts	1 oz (28g)	15	<1	4g
Pistachio Butter	2 tbsp (32g)	15	<1	4g
Pistachios	1 oz (28g)	15	<1	5g
Poppy seeds	1 oz (28g)	5	<1	2g
Poppy seeds	1 oz (28g)	5	<1	3g
Pumpkin seeds (Pepitas)	1 oz (28g)	15	<1	2g
Quinoa seeds	1 oz (28g)	53	2.2	4g
Raw Almonds	1 oz (28g)	0	0	2g
Raw Brazil Nuts	1 oz (28g)	15	0	1g
Raw Cashews	1 oz (28g)	25	2	8g
Raw Chia Nuts	1 oz (28g)	5	<1	1g
Raw Hazelnuts (Filberts)	1 oz (28g)	15	<1	2g
Raw Macadamia Nuts	1 oz (28g)	15	<1	2g
Raw Peanuts	1 oz (28g)	13	<1	3g
Raw Pecans	1 oz (28g)	0	0	1g
Raw Pine Nuts	1 oz (28g)	15	<1	4g
Raw Pistachios	1 oz (28g)	15	<1	5g
Raw Walnuts	1 oz (28g)	15	<1	1g
Roasted Almonds	1 oz (28g)	0	0	2g
Roasted Brazil Nuts	1 oz (28g)	15	<1	1g
Roasted Cashews	1 oz (28g)	25	2	8g
Roasted Chestnuts	1 oz (28g)	60	8	14g
Roasted Chia Nuts	1 oz (28g)	1	<1	1g
Roasted Hazelnuts	1 oz (28g)	15	<1	2g

NUTS & SEEDS	SERVING SIZE	GI	GL	NET CARB
Roasted Macadamia Nuts	1 oz (28g)	15	<1	2g
Roasted Peanuts	1 oz (28g)	13	<1	3g
Roasted Pecans	1 oz (28g)	0	0	1g
Roasted Pine Nuts	1 oz (28g)	15	<1	4g
Roasted Pistachios	1 oz (28g)	15	<1	5g
Roasted Walnuts	1 oz (28g)	15	<1	1g
Salted Almonds	1 oz (28g)	0	0	2g
Salted Brazil Nuts	1 oz (28g)	15	<1	1g
Salted Cashews	1 oz (28g)	25	2	8g
Salted Hazelnuts	1 oz (28g)	15	<1	2g
Salted Macadamia Nuts	1 oz (28g)	15	<1	2g
Salted Peanuts	1 oz (28g)	13	<1	3g
Salted Pecans	1 oz (28g)	0	0	1g
Salted Pistachios	1 oz (28g)	15	<1	5g
Salted Walnuts	1 oz (28g)	15	<1	1g
Sesame seeds	1 oz (28g)	35	1	3g
Sesame seeds	1 oz (28g)	35	1	3g
Steamed Chestnuts	1 oz (28g)	60	8	14g
Sunflower seeds	1 oz (28g)	15	<1	3g
Tiger nuts	1 oz (28g)	51	6	11g
Walnut Oil	1 tbsp (14g)	0	0	0g
Walnuts	1 oz (28g)	15	<1	1g
Watermelon seeds	1 oz (28g)	10	<1	1g

OIL AND CONDIMENTS

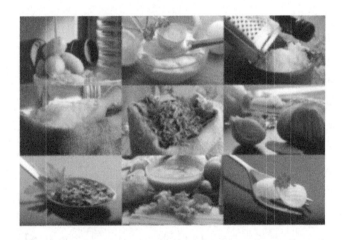

As you navigate through the journey of reversing Type 2 Diabetes (T2D), you will find that the right choices in oils and condiments can make a profound difference. Fats are not merely an indispensable part of our diet but also crucial for many body functions. Likewise, condiments, while used in small quantities, can contribute significantly to the taste, enjoyment, and nutritional value of our meals.

Compliant Oils and Fats:

When it comes to fats and oils, it's not just the quantity that counts, but the quality too. To support T2D reversal, focusing on unsaturated fats is essential, which can help improve heart health and blood glucose control.

- **Olive Oil:** Rich in monounsaturated fats, olive oil can help lower bad LDL cholesterol and improve insulin sensitivity. Choose extra virgin olive oil for maximum health benefits.
- **Avocado Oil:** Avocado oil shares similarities with olive oil, as it contains abundant heart-healthy monounsaturated fats. Additionally, it possesses a high smoke point, allowing for safe usage in high-temperature cooking.
- **Canola Oil:** This is another great option, offering a balance of monounsaturated and polyunsaturated fats. It also has a high smoke point, making it suitable for various cooking methods.
- **Flaxseed Oil:** Flaxseed oil is widely acknowledged as a potent and excellent source of omega-3, which aid in the reduction of inflammation. However, due to its low smoke point, it's best used in cold dishes like salads.
- **Nuts and Seeds:** Almonds, walnuts, flaxseeds, and chia seeds are abundant in beneficial fats, fiber, and protein, making them a nutritious addition to one's diet.
- **Fatty Fish:** Salmon, mackerel, sardines, and trout are excellent sources of omega-3 fatty acids, promoting heart health and reducing inflammation.

Remember to consider cooking methods too. Opt for grilling, roasting, steaming, and sautéing over deep frying to avoid the formation of harmful compounds.

Compliant Condiments:

Selecting condiments wisely can help you avoid hidden sugars, unhealthy fats, and excessive sodium, which are not beneficial for T2D management.

- **Mustard:** Pure mustard, especially Dijon or whole-grain variants, is a good low-sugar and low-calorie choice.
- **Vinegar:** Apple cider vinegar, balsamic vinegar, and other vinegars can add a flavorful tang without spiking your blood sugar levels.
- **Salsa:** Fresh salsa made from tomatoes, onions, cilantro, and peppers is a nutrient-rich, low-calorie option.
- **Herbs and Spices:** Fresh or dried herbs and spices like rosemary, thyme, oregano, garlic, and turmeric can add a burst of flavor without extra calories or sugars.
- **Homemade Dressings:** By making your own salad dressings with compliant oils, vinegar, herbs, and spices, you control the ingredients, avoiding added sugars and unhealthy fats.
- **Sugar-free or Low-sodium Sauces:** When purchasing store-bought condiments, look for sugar-free or low-sodium versions to better align with your Reverse Type 2 Diabetes Diet.

By paying attention to the quality and sources of fats and condiments, you can enhance the flavor of your meals while supporting your efforts to reverse T2D. It is important to approach these elements with moderation, considering portion sizes and closely monitoring how different foods impact your blood sugar levels. Being mindful of your choices regarding fats and condiments can contribute to a balanced and effective Reverse Type 2 Diabetes Diet.

The following section of this chapter presents comprehensive tables of foods that are fully compliant with Reverse Type 2 Diabetes Diet. Each entry is accompanied by crucial information such as serving size, Glycemic Index (GI), Glycemic Load (GL), and Net Carbohydrates, enabling the reader to make informed decisions about portion sizes and meal planning.

However, it's important to note that not all compliant foods are equal. Some foods, while fitting within the parameters of the Reverse Type 2 Diabetes Diet, are more beneficial than others. For instance, foods that are minimally processed, lower in sodium, and rich in healthy fats are preferable. For these food items, even though GI, GL, and net carb data might not be the sole determinants of their suitability, their overall nutritional profile makes them excellent choices.

This distinction between different compliant foods enhances clarity and helps readers understand why certain foods are more desirable within the framework of the Reverse Type 2 Diabetes Diet. It also guides readers towards making healthier choices that align with the principles of this dietary approach and contribute to sustainable and effective diabetes management.

MEDITERRANEAN RESTAURANT FOODS

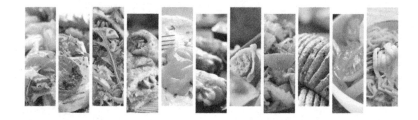

Mediterranean cuisine, renowned for its emphasis on plant-based foods, healthy fats, and lean proteins, holds a prominent position in diets worldwide. This includes the diets of individuals seeking to manage or reverse Type 2 diabetes. However, the suitability of these Mediterranean foods for a Reverse Type 2 Diabetes Diet hinges on several factors such as their Glycemic Load (GL), nutritional content, and overall dietary compatibility. Gaining a comprehensive understanding of the advantages and possible drawbacks of Mediterranean foods is essential for making informed decisions about dietary choices that can effectively support diabetes management and promote overall health.

Benefits of Mediterranean Foods:

- **Nutrient-Dense:** Mediterranean foods are traditionally rich in vital nutrients, including dietary fiber, vitamins, and minerals. This cuisine underscores the importance of fresh fruits and vegetables, lean proteins, whole grains, and healthy fats, contributing to its nutrient-rich profile.
- **Heart-Healthy:** The Mediterranean diet is often linked with improved heart health, largely due to its focus on healthy fats from sources such as olive oil and fish. These fats are known to support heart health by reducing levels of harmful cholesterol and providing essential fatty acids.
- **Low Glycemic Load:** A significant proportion of traditional Mediterranean foods have a low glycemic load. This means they impact blood sugar levels minimally, making them particularly suitable for individuals with Type 2 diabetes.

Potential Drawbacks of Mediterranean Foods:

- **High in Carbohydrates:** Certain Mediterranean foods, notably specific types of bread and pasta, have high carbohydrate content. These foods can cause abrupt rise in blood sugar levels if not portioned correctly. Some non-compliant examples include migas, pita bread, Moroccan couscous, and the Serranito sandwich, primarily due to their high carbohydrate content.
- **Cooking Methods and Ingredients:** Some Mediterranean dishes may utilize cooking techniques or ingredients that aren't in line with a Reverse Type 2 Diabetes Diet. It is essential to scrutinize both the ingredients list and the preparation methods when selecting dishes to incorporate into your diet. Fried foods and those with added sugars are examples of potentially problematic foods within Mediterranean cuisine.

* * *

The following section of this chapter presents comprehensive tables of foods that are fully compliant with Reverse Type 2 Diabetes Diet. Each entry is accompanied by crucial information such as serving size, Glycemic Index (GI), Glycemic Load (GL), and Net Carbohydrates, enabling the reader to make informed decisions about portion sizes and meal planning.

However, it's important to note that not all compliant foods are equal. Some foods, while fitting within the parameters of the Reverse Type 2 Diabetes Diet, are more beneficial than others. For instance, foods that are minimally processed, lower in sodium, and rich in healthy fats are preferable. For these food items, even though GI, GL, and net carb data might not be the sole determinants of their suitability, their overall nutritional profile makes them excellent choices.

This distinction between different compliant foods enhances clarity and helps readers understand why certain foods are more desirable within the framework of the Reverse Type 2 Diabetes Diet. It also guides readers towards making healthier choices that align with the principles of this dietary approach and contribute to sustainable and effective diabetes management.

MEDITERRANEAN RESTAURANT FOODS

MEDITERRANEAN RESTAURANT FOOD	SERVING SIZE	GI	GL	NET CARB
Ajoblanco	1 cup (250g)	30	4.5	15g
Almond Gazpacho	1 cup (250g)	30	3	10g
Baba Ganoush	2 tbsp (30g)	15	0.6	4g
Bouillabaisse	1 bowl (250g)	15	1.1	7g
Calamari	1 serving (150g)	40	4	10g
Caldo Gallego	1 bowl (250g)	30	4.5	15g
Caponata	1 cup (200g)	40	8	20g
Caprese Salad	1 serving (150g)	15	0.8	5g
Chicken Souvlaki	1 skewer (85g)	0	0	0g
Cocido Madrileno	1 serving (400g)	40	10	25g
Croquetas	1 croqueta (30g)	50	5	10g
Dolmades (grape leaves)	1 dolmade (30g)	35	3.5	10g
Eggplant Parmigiana	1 serving (200g)	35	7	20g
Escalivada	1 serving (150g)	15	1.5	10g
Espinacas con garbanzos	1 serving (150g)	35	5.2	15g
Fabada Asturiana	½ bowl (150g)	40	4	10g
Fabes con Almejas	1 serving (150g)	35	3.5	10g
Falafel	1 piece (17g)	52	2.6	5g
Feta Cheese	1 ounce (28g)	0	0	1g
Gambas al Ajillo	1 serving (150g)	10	0.3	3g
Gambas Pil Pil	1 serving (150g)	5	0.1	2g
Gazpacho	1 cup (250g)	35	5.3	15g
Greek Egg-Lemon Soup (Avgolemono)	1 cup (245g)	20	3	15g
Greek Fava	½ cup (85g)	35	4.4	12.5g

MEDITERRANEAN RESTAURANT FOOD	SERVING SIZE	GI	GL	NET CARB
Greek Salad	1 cup (100g)	15	0.8	5g
Greek Yogurt (plain)	1 cup (245g)	15	1.1	7g
Grilled Octopus	1 serving (150g)	0	0	0g
Gyro (without bread)	1 gyro (200g)	10	0.8	8g
Halloumi Cheese	1 ounce (28g)	0	0	1g
Huevos Rotos	1 serving (150g)	30	5	15g
Hummus	2 tbsp (30g)	6	0.5	8g
Imam Bayildi (stuffed eggplant)	½ piece (200g)	35	3.5	10g
Italian Antipasto	1 serving (150g)	20	2	10g
Jamon Iberico	2 slices (30g)	0	0	0g
Kofta	1 piece (100g)	10	0.5	5g
Labneh	2 tbsp (30g)	20	0.6	3g
Lamb Kofta	1 piece (100g)	10	0.5	5g
Lamb Souvlaki	1 skewer (85g)	0	0	0g
Lentil Soup	½ bowl (125g)	30	4.5	15g
Marinated olives	10 olives (40g)	0	0	0g
Mariscada	1 serving (300g)	0	0	0g
Mediterranean Chicken	1 serving (200g)	0	0	0g
Melitzanosalata	2 tbsp (30g)	15	0.6	4g
Morcilla	1 link (75g)	5	0.2	3g
Moussaka	1 piece (200g)	40	4	10g
Olive Tapenade	2 tbsp (30g)	20	0.4	2g
Paella (without rice)	1 serving (250g)	25	3.8	15g
Pan con Tomate	1 serving (70g)	60	9	15g
Pimientos de Padrón	10 peppers (80g)	10	0.5	5g
Pincho Moruno	1 pincho (100g)	0	0	0g
Piquillo peppers stuffed	1 pepper (50g)	20	1.2	6g
Pisto	1 cup (200g)	35	5.3	15g

MEDITERRANEAN RESTAURANT FOOD	SERVING SIZE	GI	GL	NET CARB
Pollo al Ajillo	1 serving (200g)	0	0	2g
Prawn Saganaki	1 serving (200g)	5	0.4	8g
Pulpo a la Gallega	1 serving (150g)	20	1	5g
Queso Manchego	1 ounce (28g)	0	0	0g
Rabo de Toro	1 serving (250g)	0	0	3g
Ratatouille	1 cup (200g)	35	5.3	15g
Saganaki	1 serving (100g)	15	0.3	2g
Salmorejo	1 cup (250g)	30	4.5	15g
Shakshuka	1 serving (250g)	25	3.8	15g
Sobrassada	2 slices (30g)	0	0	0g
Spanakopita	1 piece (85g)	40	4	10g
Spanish Bean Soup (Cocido)	½ bowl (125g)	30	3	10g
Spanish Blue Cheese	1 ounce (28g)	0	0	0g
Spanish omelette	1 serving (150g)	25	3.8	15g
Tabouli Salad	½ cup (75g)	35	3.5	10g
Tapas (mixed)	1 serving (100g)	30	3	10g
Taramasalata	2 tbsp (30g)	15	0.5	3g
Turkish Delight	1 piece (10g)	65	6.5	10g
Turkish Menemen	1 serving (200g)	15	1.5	10g
Tzatziki	2 tbsp (30g)	15	0.5	3g
Zarzuela de Mariscos	1 serving (300g)	10	0.8	8g

VEGETABLES AND VEGETABLE PRODUCTS

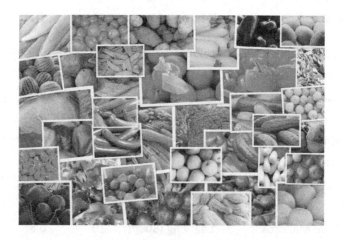

Vegetables and vegetable products play a key role in numerous diets around the world, and they're integral to the dietary regimen of those pursuing a type 2 diabetes (T2D) reversal diet. Assessing their glycemic load (GL), nutritional content, and suitability for a Reverse Type 2 Diabetes Diet is crucial. Understanding the advantages and potential pitfalls of vegetables and vegetable products can guide individuals to make informed dietary choices, promoting diabetes management and overall health.

Benefits of Vegetables and Vegetable Products:

- **Nutrient-Dense:** Vegetables are packed with an array of essential nutrients, such as vitamins, minerals, trace minerals, dietary fiber, and antioxidants, contributing to overall health and well-being.
- **Low in Calories:** Most vegetables are low in calories, making them a favorable choice for weight management.
- **High in Fiber:** Vegetables are an excellent source of dietary fiber, which delays the absorption of sugar into your bloodstream, helping prevent abrupt increases in blood glucose and insulin levels.

JUICES, HIGH SODIUM PREPARATIONS, AND COOKING METHODS:

Fruit and Vegetable Juices: While fruit and vegetable juices can provide nutrients, they often lack the dietary fiber found naturally in whole fruits and vegetables. They are also high in sugar, quickly raising blood sugar levels. Therefore, it's generally better to consume whole fruits and vegetables instead of their juiced counterparts.

High Sodium Preparations: Some canned or pre-packaged vegetables are high in sodium, which can be harmful, particularly for individuals with high blood pressure, and increases the risk of devastating complications. Always check the nutrition label to choose low-sodium or no-salt-added options whenever possible.

Cooking Methods: The way vegetables are prepared can affect their nutritional value. Some cooking methods, such as deep frying, add a substantial amount of fat and calories. Others, like boiling, can leach water-soluble nutrients. Healthier cooking methods, such as steaming, sautéing, grilling, roasting, or eating vegetables raw, can help maintain their nutrient content and keep added fat to a minimum.

Incorporating these factors into your Reverse Type 2 Diabetes Diet can aid in making healthier choices. This diet emphasizes the importance of whole, unprocessed foods and minimally added sugars, sodium, and unhealthy fats. Recognizing how preparation and cooking methods can alter the nutritional profile of vegetables is vital to managing diabetes effectively.

Potential Drawbacks of Vegetables and Vegetable Products:

- **Starchy Vegetables:** Some vegetables, particularly starchy ones like potatoes, corn, and peas, can be higher in carbohydrates and may raise blood glucose levels if not consumed in moderation.
- **Processed Vegetable Products:** Certain processed vegetable products, like canned vegetables or vegetable juices, may contain added sugars, sodium, or other additives, making them less ideal for those managing diabetes.

Incorporating Vegetables and Vegetable Products into your eating plan:

- **Emphasize Non-Starchy Vegetables:** Non-starchy vegetables, such as leafy greens, broccoli, bell peppers, and zucchini, have fewer carbs than their starchy counterparts and can be consumed in larger quantities.
- **Monitor Portion Sizes:** Although vegetables are generally healthy, portion control is particularly important for starchy vegetables due to their higher carbohydrate content.
- **Choose Fresh or Frozen Over Canned:** Fresh or frozen vegetables are usually healthier than canned ones, which often contain added sodium. If choosing canned vegetables, look for low-sodium or no-salt-added versions.
- **Read Labels Diligently:** Pay careful attention to labels when purchasing vegetable products. Aim for products with minimal added sugars, sodium, or other additives.

* * *

The following section of this chapter presents comprehensive tables of foods that are fully compliant with Reverse Type 2 Diabetes Diet. Each entry is accompanied by crucial information such as serving size, Glycemic Index (GI), Glycemic Load (GL), and Net Carbohydrates, enabling the reader to make informed decisions about portion sizes and meal planning.

However, it's important to note that not all compliant foods are equal. Some foods, while fitting within the parameters of the Reverse Type 2 Diabetes Diet, are more beneficial than others. For instance, foods that are minimally processed, lower in sodium, and rich in healthy fats are preferable. For these food items, even though GI, GL, and net carb data might not be the sole determinants of their suitability, their overall nutritional profile makes them excellent choices.

This distinction between different compliant foods enhances clarity and helps readers understand why certain foods are more desirable within the framework of the Reverse Type 2 Diabetes Diet. It also guides readers towards making healthier choices that align with the principles of this dietary approach and contribute to sustainable and effective diabetes management.

VEGETABLES & VEGETABLE PRODUCTS

VEGETABLES & VEGETABLE PRODUCTS	SERVING SIZE	GI	GL	NET CARB
LOW GLYCEMIC LOAD FOODS				
Alfalfa Sprouts	1 cup (33g)	15	1	0.4g
Amaranth Leaves Cooked Boiled With Salt Drained	1 cup (132g)	65	4	5.4g
Amaranth Leaves Cooked Boiled Without Salt Drained	1 cup (132g)	65	4	5.4g
Artichoke Dip	2 tbsp (30g)	15	1	2g
Artichoke Hearts	1 cup (168g)	20	5	12g
Artichoke	1 medium (120g)	20	3	9g
Artichokes, (globe or french), raw	1 medium (120g)	15-20	4	4.2g
Arugula, raw	1 cup (20g)	20-30	0	0.4g
Asparagus Chips	1 oz (28g)	15	1	7g
Asparagus Pea	1 cup (90g)	15-20	1	4g
Asparagus Puree	1/2 cup (125g)	15	1	4g
Asparagus	1 cup (134g)	15	1	4g
Avocado	1/2 avocado (100g)	15	0	2g
Baba Ghanoush	2 tbsp (30g)	15	1	3g
Balsam-pear (bitter gourd), leafy tips, raw	1 cup (64g)	15-25	1	1.6g
Balsam-pear (bitter gourd), pods, raw	1 cup (93g)	15-25	1	2.3g
Bamboo Shoots	1 cup (151g)	15	1	3g
Bean Sprouts	1 cup (104g)	30	2	4g
Beans, fava, in pod, raw	1 cup (130g)	20-30	2	7.8g

VEGETABLES & VEGETABLE PRODUCTS	SERVING SIZE	GI	GL	NET CARB
Beans, kidney, mature seeds, soaked and cooked	1 cup (104g)	25-40	3	3.7g
Beans, navy, mature seeds, soaked and cooked	1 cup (104g)	20-30	1	2.8g
Beans, pinto, mature seeds, soaked and cooked	1 cup (104g)	25-40	2	5.5g
Beans, snap, green, soaked and cooked	1 cup (100g)	20-Oct	1	3.9g
Beans, snap, yellow, , soaked and cooked	1 cup (100g)	20-30	1	3.2g
Beet Chips	1 oz (28g)	61	5	11g
Beet Greens, Cooked with salt	1 cup (144g)	15	1	3g
Beet Greens, Cooked without salt	1 cup (144g)	15	1	3g
Beet Greens, Raw,	1 cup (144g)	15	1	3g
Beetroot Powder	1 tbsp (8g)	61	2	5g
Beetroot Puree	1/2 cup (125g)	61	7	14g
Beets Cooked Boiled. Drained With Salt	1 cup (136g)	60-70	5	13g
Beets, cooked without salt	1 cup (136g)	64	7	13g
Beets, raw	1 cup (136g)	60-70	5	13g
Bell Peppers	1 cup (149g)	15	1	6g
Bitter Melon, Cooked with salt	1/2 cup (100g)	15-30	3	4g
Bitter Melon	1/2 cup (100g)	15-30	3	4g
Black Beans	1 cup (172g)	30	8	24g
Bok Choy, Cooked	1 cup (170g)	15	0	1g
Bok Choy, Raw	1 cup (170g)	15	0	1g
Borage Cooked Boiled Drained With Salt	1 cup (89g)	15-20	1	0.6g
Borage Cooked Boiled Drained Without Salt	1 cup (89g)	15-20	1	0.6g

VEGETABLES & VEGETABLE PRODUCTS	SERVING SIZE	GI	GL	NET CARB
Borage, raw	1 cup (89g)	15-20	1	0.6g
Broccoflower Cooked	1 cup (100g)	15	1	3g
Broccoflower, Raw	1 cup (100g)	15	1	3g
Broccoli Powder	1 tbsp (7g)	15	1	4.4g
Broccoli Puree	1/2 cup (125g)	15	1	6g
Broccoli raab, raw	1 cup (40g)	15-20	1	0.7g
Broccoli Stem Noodles	1 cup (100g)	15	1	3g
Broccoli, Chinese, raw	1 cup (56g)	15-20	1	1.8g
Broccoli, leaves, raw	1 cup (50g)	15-20	1	1.4g
Broccoli	1 cup (156g)	15	1	6g
Broccoli, stalks, raw	1 cup (92g)	15-20	1	3.3g
Brussels Sprouts Chips	1 oz (28g)	15	1	7g
Brussels Sprouts, Cooked	1 cup (156g)	15	2	8g
Burdock root, Cooked without salt	1 cup (116g)	40-50	7	14.3g
Burdock root, raw	1 cup (116g)	40-50	7	14.3g
Burdock, Cooked, Boiled with salt	1 cup (116g)	40-50	7	14.3g
Butterbur (fuki), raw	1 cup (55g)	15-20	1	1.5g
Butternut Squash Noodles	1 cup (150g)	51	5	13g
Butternut Squash Puree	1/2 cup (125g)	51	7	14g
Butternut Squash	1 cup (205g)	51	8	21g
Cabbage Green, Cooked without salt	1 cup (205g)	15	1	4g
Cabbage, chinese (pak-choi), raw	1 cup (70g)	15-20	1	1g
Cabbage, chinese (pe-tsai), cooked without salt	1 cup (76g)	15-20	1	1.2g
Cabbage, chinese (pe-tsai), raw	1 cup (76g)	15-20	1	1.2g
Cabbage, raw	1 cup (89g)	15-20	1	3g

VEGETABLES & VEGETABLE PRODUCTS	SERVING SIZE	GI	GL	NET CARB
Cabbage, red, raw	1 cup (89g)	15-20	1	4g
Cabbage, savoy, raw	1 cup (70g)	15-20	1	2.5g
Canned Acorn Squash	1 cup (245g)	15	1	7g
Canned Artichoke Hearts	1 cup (168g)	15	2	8g
Canned Asparagus	1 cup (200g)	15	1	6g
Canned Bamboo Shoots	1 cup (151g)	15	1	5g
Canned butternut Squash	1 cup (245g)	15	1	7g
Canned Carrots	1 cup (236g)	39	7	18g
Canned Green Beans	1 cup (240g)	15	3	12g
Canned Lima Beans	1 cup (240g)	20	5	12g
Canned Mixed Vegetables	1 cup (240g)	45	7	16g
Canned Mushrooms	1 cup (156g)	15	1	4g
Canned Okra	1 cup (256g)	15	1	4g
Canned Olives	1 ounce (28g)	15	0	1g
Canned Pickles	1 spear (35g)	15	0	1g
Canned Pumpkin	1 cup (245g)	15	3	12g
Canned Sauerkraut	1 cup (142g)	15	1	4g
Canned Spaghetti Squash	1 cup (245g)	15	1	7g
Canned Spinach	1 cup (214g)	15	1	4g
Canned Tomatoes	1 cup (240g)	45	6	13g
Canned Water Chestnuts	1 cup (140g)	54	7	14g
Cardoon Cooked Boiled with salt and drained	1 cup (150g)	15-20	1	3.5g
Cardoon Cooked Boiled with salt and drained	1 cup (150g)	15-20	1	3.5g
Cardoon, raw	1 cup (120g)	15-20	1	3.5g
Carrot Chips	1 oz (28g)	47	4	9g
Carrot Greens	1 cup (25g)	15	0	1g
Carrot Noodles	1 cup (110g)	47	4	8g

VEGETABLES & VEGETABLE PRODUCTS	SERVING SIZE	GI	GL	NET CARB
Carrot Powder	1 tbsp (7g)	47	1	3g
Carrot Puree	1/2 cup (125g)	47	7	14g
Carrot Spread	2 tbsp (30g)	35	2	4g
Carrots Cooked Boiled Drained With Salt	1 cup (128g)	39	5	13g
Carrots, baby, raw	1 cup (128g)	45-55	6	11.5g
Carrots, Cooked Boiled Drained Without Salt	1 cup (128g)	39	5	13g
Cauliflower Cooked With Salt, Boiled and Drained	1 cup (56g)	15	1	2g
Cauliflower Frozen Unprepared	1 cup (56g)	15	1	2g
Cauliflower Green Cooked With Salt	1 cup (56g)	15	1	2g
Cauliflower Greens	1 cup (56g)	15	1	2g
Cauliflower Powder	1 tbsp (6g)	15	0	1g
Cauliflower Puree	1/2 cup (125g)	15	1	4g
Celeriac Cooked Boiled With Salt Drained	1/2 cup (125g)	15	1	6g
Celeriac Cooked without salt	1 cup (156g)	15	2	9g
Celeriac Puree	1/2 cup (125g)	15	1	6g
Celeriac	1 cup (156g)	15	1	6g
Celery Powder	1 tbsp (6g)	15	0	1g
Celery Root Puree	1/2 cup (125g)	15	1	6g
Celery	1 cup (101g)	15	0	2g
Chard Cooked	1 cup (175g)	15	1	5g
Chayote Cooked Boiled with salt Drained	1 cup (132g)	15	1	4g
Chayote Fruit Raw	1 cup (132g)	15	1	4g
Chickpeas	½ cup (82g)	28	4	13.5g
Chicory greens, raw	1 cup (55g)	15-20	1	0.5g

VEGETABLES & VEGETABLE PRODUCTS	SERVING SIZE	GI	GL	NET CARB
Chicory roots, raw	1 cup (60g)	20-25	1	4g
Chicory, witloof, raw	1 cup (50g)	15-20	1	0.8g
Chives	1 tbsp (3g)	15	0	0g
Chrysanthemum leaves, raw	1 cup (43g)	15-20	1	0.6g
Chrysanthemum, garland, Cooked Boiled With Salt Drained	1 cup (20g)	15-20	1	1.2g
Collard Greens, Cooked	1 cup (190g)	15	1	5g
Collards Chopped Unprepared	1 cup (190g)	15	1	5g
Cornsalad, raw	1 cup (56g)	15-20	1	1.5g
Cowpeas, leafy tips, raw	1 cup (36g)	15-20	1	1g
Cowpeas, young pods with seeds, raw	1 cup (100g)	35-40	4	8g
Cress Garden Cooked Boiled With Salt Drained	1 cup (25g)	15-20	1	0.7g
Cress, garden, raw	1 cup (25g)	15-20	1	0.7g
Cucumber Chips	1 oz (28g)	15	1	6g
Cucumber Noodles	1 cup (100g)	15	0	2g
Cucumber, peeled, raw	1 cup (133g)	15	1	2.5g
Cucumber	1 cup (104g)	15	0	2g
Cucumber, with peel, raw	1 cup (104g)	15	1	3g
Daikon Radish Noodles	1 cup (120g)	15	1	3g
Daikon	1 cup (116g)	15	1	4g
Dandelion Greens Cooked Boiled With Salt Drained	1 cup (55g)	15	1	3g
Dandelion Greens, Cooked without salt	1 cup (55g)	15	1	3g
Dandelion Greens, Raw	1 cup (55g)	15	1	3g
Dock, raw	1 cup (133g)	15-20	1	2g

VEGETABLES & VEGETABLE PRODUCTS	SERVING SIZE	GI	GL	NET CARB
Drumstick Leaves Cooked Boiled Drained With Salt	1/2 cup (100g)	15-20	1	0.5g
Drumstick Leaves Cooked Boiled Drained Without Salt	1/2 cup (100g)	15-20	1	0.5g
Drumstick leaves, raw	1 cup (21g)	15-20	1	0.5g
Drumstick pods, raw	1 cup (99g)	20-25	2	4g
Edamame Cooked	1 cup (155g)	15	3	8g
Edamame Unprepared	1/2 cup (75g)	15	3	8g
Eggplant Noodles	1 cup (100g)	15	0	2g
Eggplant, Raw	1 cup (99g)	15	1	6g
Endive Leaves	1 cup (40g)	15	0	1g
Endive	1 cup (50g)	15	0	1g
Epazote, raw	1 cup (20g)	15-20	1	0.7g
Eppaw, raw	1 cup (20g)	15-20	1	1g
Escarole Cooked without salt	1 cup (75g)	15	1	3g
Escarole Creamed	1 cup (75g)	15	1	3g
Fennel Bulb Cooked Boiled with salt drained	1 cup (87g)	15	1	5g
Fennel Puree	½ cup (125g)	15	1	5g
Fennel Sliced Serving size 1 cup (87g): GI of 15	1 cup (87g)	15	1	4g
Fiddlehead ferns, raw	1 cup (87g)	15-20	1	4g
Fireweed, leaves, raw	1 cup (35g)	15-20	1	1.5g
Garlic Powder	1 teaspoon (3g)	15	0	1g
Garlic Scapes	1 cup (40g)	15	0	1g
Garlic	1 clove (3g)	15	0	1g
Ginger root, raw	1 tbsp (9g)	15-20	1	1g
Ginger	1 tbsp (6g)	15	0	1g

VEGETABLES & VEGETABLE PRODUCTS	SERVING SIZE	GI	GL	NET CARB
Gourd, dishcloth (towelgourd), raw	1 cup (86g)	15-20	1	2g
Gourd, white-flowered (calabash), raw	1 cup (116g)	15-20	1	3g
Grape Leaves Canned	1 cup (28g)	15-20	1	1.5g
Grape leaves, raw	1 cup (28g)	15-20	1	1.5g
Green Bean Chips	1 oz (28g)	15	1	6g
Green Beans	1 cup (125g)	15	1	5g
Green Bell Pepper Powder	1 tbsp (6g)	15	0	2g
Green Onion	1 cup (100g)	15	1	4g
Guacamole	2 tbsp (30g)	15	1	2g
Hearts of palm, raw	1 cup (146g)	15-20	1	4g
Hubbard Squash	1 cup (205g)	50	6	16g
Hummus	2 tbsp (30g)	25	2	4g
Jalapeno	1 pepper (14g)	15	0	1g
Jerusalem Artichoke, Cooked	½ cup (75g)	50	3	11g
Jerusalem Artichokes Raw	½ cup (150g)	50	3	11g
Jicama Chips	1 oz (28g)	15	1	6g
Jicama Noodles	1 cup (120g)	15	2	5g
Jicama	1 cup (120g)	15	2	6g
Jute, potherb, raw	1 cup (28g)	15-20	1	0.5g
Kale Chips	1 oz (28g)	15	1	6g
Kale Cooked Boiled With Salt Drained	1 cup (130g)	15	1	4g
Kale Cooked Boiled Without Salt Drained	1 cup (130g)	15	1	4g
Kale Powder	1 tbsp (6g)	15	0	1g
Kale	1 cup (130g)	15	1	4g
Kelp	1 cup (76g)	15	0	1g

VEGETABLES & VEGETABLE PRODUCTS	SERVING SIZE	GI	GL	NET CARB
Kohlrabi Noodles	1 cup (135g)	15	1	5g
Kohlrabi	1 cup (135g)	15	2	8g
Lambsquarters, raw	1 cup (28g)	15-20	1	1g
Leek Leaves	1 cup (72g)	15	1	4g
Lemon grass (citronella), raw	1 tbsp (6g)	15-20	1	0.4g
Lemon Juice with Cayenne Pepper and Turmeric	1 cup (240ml)	22	2	6g
Lentils Sprouted Cooked Stir-Fried With Salt	1 cup (198g)	29	7	27g
Lentils Sprouts	½ cup (98g)	29	3.5	13.5g
Lettuce, green leaf, raw	1 cup (36g)	15	1	1g
Lettuce, iceberg (includes crisphead types), raw	1 cup (72g)	15	1	1g
Lettuce, red leaf, raw	1 cup (28g)	15	1	0.7g
Lettuce, Romaine	1 cup (72g)	15	0	1g
Lotus Root	1 cup (120g)	60	7	16g
Mung Bean Sprouts	1 cup (104g)	30	2	4g
Mung Beans Mature Seeds Sprouted Cooked Stir-Fried	1 cup (104g)	30	2	4g
Mung Beans, Sprouted Cooked Boiled With Salt Drained	1 cup (104g)	30	2	4g
Mung Beans, Sprouted Cooked Boiled Without Salt Drained	1 cup (104g)	30	2	4g
Mushroom Powder	1 tbsp (7g)	15	0	1g
Mushroom	1 cup (70g)	15	0	2g
Mushrooms (Portobello, Shiitake, etc.)	1 cup (86g)	15	0	2g

VEGETABLES & VEGETABLE PRODUCTS	SERVING SIZE	GI	GL	NET CARB
Mustard Spinach (Tendergreen) Cooked Boiled With Salt Drained	1 cup (140g)	15-20	1	1.5g
Mustard spinach (tendergreen), raw	1 cup (56g)	15-20	1	1.5g
Napa Cabbage	1 cup (109g)	15	1	3g
New Zealand spinach, raw	1 cup (56g)	15-20	1	1g
Nopales	1 cup (86g)	15	1	3g
Okra	1 cup (100g)	15	1	4g
Olives, Black	1 ounce (28g)	15	0	1g
Olives, Green	1 ounce (28g)	15	0	1g
Onion Cooked	1 cup (160g)	15	4	15g
Onion Juice	1 tbsp (15ml)	15	0	1g
Onion Powder	1 teaspoon (2g)	15	0	1g
Onions Welsh Raw	1 cup (160g)	15	4	15g
Onions, spring or scallions, raw	1 cup (100g)	30-35	3	6g
Onions, sweet, raw	1 cup (160g)	30-35	5	14g
Onions, welsh, raw	1 cup (100g)	30-35	3	7g
Parsnip	½ cup (78g)	52	6	12g
Parsley (10%) and Lemon (60%) Juice	1 cup (240ml)	15	1	7g
Parsley Juice 30%	1 cup (240ml)	15	1	6g
Parsley	1 tbsp (3g)	15	0	0g
Parsnip Puree	½ cup (125g)	52	8	20g
Pea Powder	1 tbsp (8g)	22	1	4g
Pea Puree	½ cup (125g)	45	5	16g
Peppers, hot chili, green, raw	1 pepper (14g)	30-35	1	1g
Peppers, hot chili, red, raw	1 pepper (45g)	30-35	1	2g

VEGETABLES & VEGETABLE PRODUCTS	SERVING SIZE	GI	GL	NET CARB
Peppers, Hungarian, raw	1 cup (125g)	15-20	1	5g
Peppers, jalapeno, raw	1 pepper (14g)	30-35	1	0.6g
Peppers, serrano, raw	1 pepper (18g)	30-35	1	1g
Peppers, sweet, green, raw	1 cup (149g)	15-20	2	6g
Peppers, sweet, red, raw	1 cup (149g)	15-20	2	6g
Peppers, sweet, yellow, raw	1 cup (149g)	15-20	2	6g
Pesto	1 tbsp (15g)	15	0	1g
Plantain Chips	1 oz (28g)	50	7	15g
Potato Chips	1 oz (28g)	56	8	15g
Pumpkin Cooked	1 cup (245g)	15	3	12g
Pumpkin flowers, raw	1 cup (18g)	15-20	1	0.5g
Pumpkin Juice	1 cup (240ml)	15	3	12g
Pumpkin leaves, raw	1 cup (33g)	15-20	1	0.6g
Pumpkin Powder	1 tbsp (6g)	15	0	2g
Pumpkin Puree	1/2 cup (125g)	15	2	10g
Purslane, raw	1 cup (43g)	15-20	1	0.7g
Radicchio	1 cup (40g)	15	0	1g
Radish Chips	1 oz (28g)	15	1	6g
Radish Juice	1 cup (240ml)	15	1	6g
Radish	1 cup (116g)	15	0	2g
Red Bell Pepper Powder	1 tbsp (6g)	15	0	2g
Red Cabbage Juice	1 cup (240ml)	15	1	9g
Rhubarb Cooked	1 cup (122g)	15	1	5g
Roasted Red Pepper Dip	2 tbsp (30g)	15	1	3g
Rutabaga Cooked Bolied Drained	½ cup (85g)	72	5	8g
Salsa	2 tbsp (30g)	25	1	2g

VEGETABLES & VEGETABLE PRODUCTS	SERVING SIZE	GI	GL	NET CARB
Salsify Cooked Boiled With Salt Drained	1 cup (133g)	30-35	3	8g
Salsify Cooked Boiled Without Salt Drained	1 cup (133g)	30-35	3	8g
Salsify, raw	1 cup (133g)	30-35	3	8g
Seaweed, agar, raw	1 cup (40g)	15-20	1	1g
Seaweed, irishmoss, raw	1 cup (40g)	15-20	1	2g
Seaweed, kelp, raw	1 cup (36g)	15-20	1	1g
Seaweed, laver, raw	1 cup (25g)	15-20	1	1g
Seaweed, spirulina, raw	1 tbsp (7g)	15-20	1	0.3g
Seaweed, wakame, raw	1 cup (10g)	15-20	1	0.5g
Sesbania flower, raw	1 cup (25g)	15-20	1	1g
Shallot	1 tbsp (10g)	15	0.3	2g
Snap Pea Crisps	1 oz (28g)	45	3	8g
Sorrel	1 cup (29g)	15	0	1g
Soybean sprouts	1 cup (172g)	20	3	10g
Soybeans	1 cup (172g)	20	3	10g
Spaghetti Squash	1 cup (155g)	15	1	7g
Spinach and Ginger Juice	1 cup (240ml)	15	1	7g
Spinach Chips	1 oz (28g)	15	1	6g
Spinach Cooked	1 cup (180g)	15	0.6	4g
Spinach Dip	2 tbsp (30g)	15	1	2g
Spinach Juice	1 cup (240ml)	15	1	5g
Spinach Powder	1 tbsp (7g)	15	0.1	1g
Spinach Puree	1/2 cup (125g)	15	0.1	1g
Squash Acorn, Cooked	½ cup (102g)	75	7.5	15g
Squash Butternut, Cooked	½ cup (102g)	51	8	21g
Squash Spaghetti, Cooked	1 cup (155g)	15	1	7g

VEGETABLES & VEGETABLE PRODUCTS	SERVING SIZE	GI	GL	NET CARB
Squash, winter, acorn, raw	1 cup (140g)	40-45	6	15g
Squash, winter, butternut, raw	1 cup (140g)	45-50	6	13g
Squash, winter, hubbard, raw	1 cup (116g)	40-45	5	11g
Squash, winter, spaghetti, raw	1 cup (101g)	15-20	1	5g
Sweet Potato Chips	1 oz (28g)	54	9	16g
Sweet potato leaves, raw	1 cup (28g)	15-20	1	1g
Sweet Potato Noodles	½ cup (70g)	63	4.5	11g
Sweet Potato Powder	1 tbsp (8g)	63	3	6g
Swiss Chard	1 cup (175g)	15	1	4g
Tapenade	1 tbsp (15g)	15	0	1g
Taro leaves, raw	1 cup (28g)	15-20	1	1g
Taro Root Chips	1 oz (28g)	55	7	14g
Taro shoots, raw	1 cup (84g)	15-20	1	2g
Taro, Tahitian, raw	½ cup (104g)	50-55	9	12.5g
Tomatillo	1 cup (132g)	15	1	4g
Tomato Juice	1 cup (240ml)	38	5	10g
Tomato Powder	1 tbsp (7g)	38	1	3g
Tomato Puree	1/2 cup (125g)	38	2	7g
Tomato, chopped	1 cup (180g)	15	1	5g
Turmeric Juice	1 tbsp (15ml)	15	0	1g
Turnip Noodles	1 cup (130g)	15	1	4g
Turnip	1 cup (156g)	62	4	8g
Vinespinach, (basella), raw	1 cup (44g)	15-20	1	0.8g
Wasabi, root, raw	1 tbsp (10g)	15-20	1	1g
Waterchestnuts, chinese, raw	1 cup (150g)	60	9	24g

VEGETABLES & VEGETABLE PRODUCTS	SERVING SIZE	GI	GL	NET CARB
Watercress Juice	1 cup (240ml)	15	1	4g
Watercress	1 cup (34g)	15	0	0g
Wax Beans	1 cup (125g)	15	1	5g
Wheatgrass Juice	1 ounce (30ml)	15	0	1g
Winged bean leaves, raw	1 cup (42g)	15-20	1	0.7g
Winged bean tuber, raw	1 cup (94g)	35-40	6	17g
Yardlong bean, raw	1 cup (100g)	15-20	1	5.5g
Zucchini Chips	1 oz (28g)	15	2	12g
Zucchini Juice	1 cup (240ml)	15	2	11g
Zucchini Noodles (Zoodles)	1 cup (120g)	15	2	4g
Zucchini Powder	1 tbsp (7g)	15	1	4g
Zucchini, baby (courgette), raw	1 cup (127g)	15	1	3g
Zucchini	1 cup (124g)	15	2	6g
MEDIUM GLYCEMIC LOAD FOODS (Consider reducing the serving size to stay below 15 grams of net carbs)				
Cassava, Cooked	½ cup (110g)	46	18	39g
Corn, sweet, white, raw	½ cup (82g)	60	11.4	19g
Corn, sweet, yellow, raw	½ cup (82g)	60	11.4	19g
Mountain yam, hawaii, raw	½ cup (82g)	58	11	18g
Potato, Cooked	½ cup (105g)	78	11	15g
Potatoes, flesh and skin, raw	1 medium (213g)	60-65	18	33g
Sweet Potato Puree	½ cup cup (125g)	63	12	24g
Sweet Potato, Cooked	½ cup cup (125g)	63	11.3	18g

PART V
WHAT TO AVOID: NON-COMPLIANT FOODS FOR THE TYPE 2 DIABETES REVERSAL DIET

UNDERSTANDING FOODS TO EXCLUDE IN THE T2D REVERSAL DIET

In the framework of the Reverse Type 2 Diabetes Diet, certain foods can interfere with T2D reversal efforts. To make the most effective dietary choices, it's important to understand the criteria that identify these detrimental foods:

- **High Glycemic Load (GL):** A food's GL considers both the quantity and quality of carbohydrates in a serving. High-GL foods prompt significant and swift spikes in blood glucose levels. Regular consumption of such foods can lead to insulin resistance, complicating T2D reversal.
- **Highly Processed Foods:** Even when the GL is low or medium, heavily processed foods may be harmful due to unhealthy additives, excessive salts, sugars, and unhealthy fats. These ingredients can induce weight gain and inflammation, negatively affecting blood sugar control and overall health.
- **Deviation from Mediterranean Diet Principles:** Non-compliance also includes foods that contradict the principles of the Mediterranean diet. This diet emphasizes whole or minimally processed foods—fruits, vegetables, olive oil, whole grains, lean proteins, and healthy fats. Foods that are heavily

processed, high in unhealthy fats, or nutritionally poor do not align with this diet and could undermine T2D reversal.

- **Contradiction with 2020-2025 Dietary Guidelines for Americans:** Foods that go against these guidelines are also non-compliant. The guidelines encourage the consumption of nutrient-dense foods—rich in essential vitamins, minerals, and other beneficial compounds, yet relatively low in calories. Foods high in added sugars, unhealthy fats, and sodium fall short of these standards.

Armed with this fundamental knowledge, the upcoming chapters will delve deeper into specific food categories such as vegetables, fruits and their by-products, meats, beverages, grains, and more. Each category will contain a comprehensive list of non-compliant foods, complete with their serving sizes, GI, GL, and net carb values, where relevant. Foods with a low or medium GL that contravene other core diet principles will also be included, underlining the comprehensive nature of dietary management in T2D reversal.

While the central focus of the Reverse Type 2 Diabetes Diet is avoiding non-compliant foods, the occasional indulgence in moderation is permissible, as long as portion sizes and frequencies are strictly regulated. An integral part of effective T2D management is achieving a daily GL target, ideally not exceeding 50.

Understanding portion sizes is essential, even when dining out. Ideally, choices at restaurants should align with the principles of the Mediterranean diet, paying particular attention to portion sizes and any added ingredients. Fast-food and American-style restaurants often serve meals that significantly deviate from these principles. In circumstances where options are limited, prioritize the healthiest choice available and consider either sharing the meal or saving a portion for later.

Navigating the realm of non-compliant foods can be a challenge, but with continuous effort and an informed approach, you can effectively manage this aspect of your diet. Tactics such as reading labels, planning ahead, practicing mindful eating, and making wise substitutions can assist you in overcoming these hurdles.

As you consistently make healthier choices over time, you will develop habits that support the Reverse Type 2 Diabetes Diet. Identifying compliant and non-compliant foods will become second nature. However, it's important to remember that everyone's journey is unique. It's perfectly okay to seek assistance and to take gradual steps toward your goal.

AMERICAN RESTAURANT FOODS

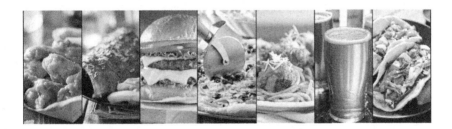

In the Reverse Type 2 Diabetes Diet, it's crucial to pay careful attention to certain American restaurant dishes that aren't aligned with its key principles, namely the Glycemic Load (GL) framework, the best practices of the Mediterranean diet (MedDiet), and the Dietary Guidelines for Americans. These dishes are typically high in carbohydrates, sugars, and unhealthy fats. When dining out, lean toward healthier options like grilled lean meats, steamed vegetables, and salads with light dressings. Additionally, choose whole grain or vegetable-based sides when possible. When healthier choices are not available, limit portion sizes. While an occasional small portion of these foods may not ruin Reverse Type 2 Diabetes Diet, they are best avoided.

DEEP-FRIED APPETIZERS

Deep-Fried Appetizers include items such as fried mozzarella sticks, onion rings, and chicken wings.

Non-Compliance with Reverse Type 2 Diabetes Diet: These foods generally do not align with the principles of the Reverse Type 2 Diabetes Diet or the 2020-2025 Dietary Guidelines for Americans.

Deep-fried appetizers are typically rich in unhealthy fats due to the frying process. This, combined with their high sodium content, can increase the risk of cardiovascular diseases - a critical concern for individuals with diabetes who need to manage their heart health vigilantly.

Moreover, these appetizers are often coated in high-carb breading, leading to unpredictable effects on blood sugar levels. The carbohydrate content can lead to significant spikes in blood sugar levels, which are particularly concerning for those seeking to manage or reverse T2D.

Additionally, these appetizers lack dietary fiber, a key nutrient in regulating blood sugar levels and supporting overall digestive health.

Furthermore, the frequent consumption of deep-fried foods can contribute to weight gain and obesity, exacerbating the challenges of managing diabetes.

Given their high content of unhealthy fats, high sodium levels, and high carbohydrate content, deep-fried appetizers are generally not recommended for individuals seeking to manage or reverse T2D. When choosing foods, it is crucial to review nutrition labels carefully and favor fresh, minimally processed foods wherever possible.

⊘ Fried artichoke hearts ⊘ Fried asparagus spears ⊘ Fried avocado slices ⊘ Fried bacon-wrapped jalapeno poppers ⊘ Fried banana peppers ⊘ Fried buffalo cauliflower ⊘

Fried calamari ⊘ Fried catfish nuggets ⊘ Fried cheese balls ⊘ Fried cheese curds ⊘ Fried cheese fries ⊘ Fried cheese-filled pretzels ⊘ Fried chicken gizzards ⊘ Fried chicken livers ⊘ Fried chicken tenders/strips ⊘ Fried chicken wings ⊘ Fried chicken-fried steak bites ⊘ Fried clam strips ⊘ Fried corn nuggets ⊘ Fried crab cakes ⊘ Fried deviled eggs ⊘ Fried dill pickle chips ⊘ Fried dumplings ⊘ Fried egg rolls ⊘ Fried green beans ⊘ Fried green tomatoes ⊘ Fried hush puppies ⊘ Fried jalapeno and cheese tater tots ⊘ Fried jalapeno bottle caps ⊘ Fried jalapeno poppers ⊘ Fried mac and cheese bites ⊘ Fried mozzarella sticks ⊘ Fried mushrooms ⊘ Fried okra ⊘ Fried oysters ⊘ Fried pickled okra ⊘ Fried pickles ⊘ Fried polenta sticks ⊘ Fried pork dumplings (potstickers) ⊘ Fried potato skins ⊘ Fried ravioli ⊘ Fried samosas ⊘ Fried shrimp ⊘ Fried spring rolls ⊘ Fried stuffed jalapenos ⊘ Fried sweet plantains ⊘ Fried turkey legs ⊘ Fried wontons ⊘ Fried zucchini sticks ⊘ Onion rings

LOADED NACHOS

Loaded Nachos, piled with cheese, sour cream, guacamole, and other high-calorie ingredients, are a common sight at many restaurants.

Non-Compliance with Reverse Type 2 Diabetes Diet: Loaded nachos typically do not align with the principles of the Reverse Type 2 Diabetes Diet or the 2020-2025 Dietary Guidelines for Americans.

These dishes are often high in both unhealthy fats and sodium due to the cheese and other toppings, contributing to increased cardiovascular disease risk - an important consideration for individuals with diabetes who need to manage their heart health carefully.

Moreover, the high carbohydrate content from the tortilla chips can lead to substantial increases in blood sugar levels, a significant concern for those managing T2D.

Loaded nachos also frequently lack sufficient dietary fiber, an essential nutrient for managing blood sugar levels and promoting overall digestive health. Additionally, their high-calorie content can contribute to weight gain and obesity, further complicating diabetes management.

Considering their high content of unhealthy fats, high sodium levels, significant carbohydrate content, and potential contribution to weight gain, loaded nachos are typically not recommended for individuals seeking to manage or reverse T2D. Making informed food choices, carefully reviewing nutrition labels, and favoring fresh, minimally processed foods are key strategies in managing diabetes.

⊘ *Classic loaded nachos with cheese, sour cream, and guacamole* ⊘ *Loaded avocado and black bean nachos* ⊘ *Loaded bacon and ranch nachos* ⊘ *Loaded BBQ chicken nachos* ⊘ *Loaded beef or steak nachos* ⊘ *Loaded BLT (bacon, lettuce, and tomato) nachos* ⊘ *Loaded breakfast nachos with eggs, bacon, and cheese* ⊘ *Loaded buffalo chicken nachos* ⊘ *Loaded buffalo ranch cauliflower nachos* ⊘ *Loaded chicken enchilada nachos* ⊘ *Loaded chili cheese nachos* ⊘ *Loaded chili dog nachos* ⊘ *Loaded chipotle chicken nachos* ⊘ *Loaded chorizo nachos* ⊘ *Loaded French fry nachos with cheese and bacon* ⊘ *Loaded Greek nachos with tzatziki sauce, feta cheese, and cucumbers* ⊘ *Loaded guacamole and pico de gallo nachos* ⊘ *Loaded Hawaiian BBQ chicken nachos* ⊘ *Loaded Hawaiian-style nachos with pineapple and ham* ⊘ *Loaded Indian-inspired nachos with curry sauce and paneer* ⊘ *Loaded Italian nachos with marinara sauce, cheese, and pepperoni* ⊘ *Loaded jalapeno popper nachos* ⊘ *Loaded Korean BBQ nachos* ⊘ *Loaded mac and cheese nachos Ⓢ Loaded Mediterranean-style nachos with feta cheese and olives Ⓢ Loaded Mexican street corn nachos Ⓢ Loaded mushroom and Swiss cheese nachos Ⓢ Loaded nachos with queso dip and salsa Ⓢ Loaded pastrami or Reuben-style nachos Ⓢ Loaded Philly cheesesteak nachos Ⓢ Loaded pulled pork nachos Ⓢ Loaded Santa Fe nachos with black beans and corn Ⓢ Loaded seafood nachos (e.g., shrimp or crab) Ⓢ Loaded spinach and artichoke dip nachos Ⓢ Loaded sweet and spicy Thai nachos Ⓢ Loaded teriyaki beef nachos Ⓢ Loaded teriyaki chicken nachos Ⓢ Loaded Tex-Mex nachos with chili, cheese, and jalapenos Ⓢ Loaded Tex-Mex nachos with pulled pork and coleslaw Ⓢ Loaded vegetarian nachos with beans, cheese, and salsa*

PASTA DISHES

Pasta Dishes, including favorites like fettuccine Alfredo or spaghetti with meatballs, are staples in many restaurants. However, these meals are often served in large portions that can significantly impact blood sugar levels.

Non-Compliance with Reverse Type 2 Diabetes Diet: Pasta dishes typically do not align with the principles of the Reverse Type 2 Diabetes Diet or the 2020-2025 Dietary Guidelines for Americans.

Pasta is a high-carbohydrate food, and a single serving can contain more carbohydrates than recommended for those managing diabetes. Especially when served in large portions, pasta can cause substantial spikes in blood sugar levels.

Furthermore, pasta dishes often come with high-fat, creamy sauces or are accompanied by meatballs or sausages, increasing the overall calorie and saturated fat content of the meal. This could contribute to weight gain and associated health risks.

These meals typically lack sufficient dietary fiber, which is crucial for managing blood sugar levels and promoting overall digestive health.

Also, the high glycemic load of pasta means that it can rapidly raise blood glucose levels, which can be particularly problematic for individuals with T2D.

Given their high carbohydrate content, potential for high fat and calorie content, low fiber, and high glycemic load, pasta dishes are typically not recommended for those managing or seeking to reverse T2D. It's crucial to make informed food choices, carefully review nutrition labels, and favor fresh, minimally processed foods when possible.

> Ⓢ *Baked ziti* Ⓢ *Fettuccine Alfredo* Ⓢ *Lasagna* Ⓢ *Macaroni and cheese* Ⓢ *Pasta primavera with creamy sauce* Ⓢ *Pasta with bacon and cream sauce* Ⓢ *Pasta with butter and Parmesan cheese* Ⓢ *Pasta with chicken and mushroom cream sauce* Ⓢ *Pasta with cream-based Marsala or wine sauce* Ⓢ *Pasta with cream-based pesto and sun-dried tomato sauce* Ⓢ *Pasta with cream-based seafood sauce* Ⓢ *Pasta with cream-based vodka or pink sauce* Ⓢ *Pasta with creamy avocado or guacamole sauce* Ⓢ *Pasta with creamy blue cheese sauce* Ⓢ *Pasta with creamy Cajun or spicy sauce* Ⓢ *Pasta with creamy caramelized onion sauce* Ⓢ *Pasta with creamy chipotle or spicy sauce* Ⓢ *Pasta with creamy curry sauce* Ⓢ *Pasta with creamy garlic sauce* Ⓢ *Pasta with creamy goat cheese sauce* Ⓢ *Pasta with creamy lemon sauce* Ⓢ *Pasta with creamy lobster or crab sauce* Ⓢ *Pasta with creamy pesto sauce* Ⓢ *Pasta with creamy mushroom sauce* Ⓢ *Pasta with creamy sausage and spinach sauce* Ⓢ *Pasta with creamy seafood or shrimp scampi sauce* Ⓢ *Pasta with creamy spinach sauce* Ⓢ *Pasta with creamy sun-dried tomato and basil sauce* Ⓢ *Pasta with creamy tomato sauce*

⊘ *Pasta with creamy truffle or mushroom truffle sauce*
⊘ *Pasta with creamy Tuscan or roasted red pepper sauce*
⊘ *Pasta with four cheese sauce* ⊘ *Pasta with meatballs or sausage in tomato sauce* ⊘ *Pasta with sausage and cream sauce* ⊘ *Pasta with shrimp scampi or buttery garlic sauce* ⊘ *Pasta with sun-dried tomato cream sauce* ⊘ *Pasta with vodka sauce* ⊘ *Pasta with white clam sauce* ⊘ *Pesto pasta* ⊘ *Spaghetti carbonara*

BREADED AND FRIED FOODS

Breaded and Fried Foods, such as breaded fish or chicken sandwiches, fried chicken tenders, and fried seafood baskets, are common menu items in many restaurants. Coated in high-carb breading and deep-fried, these foods can lead to blood sugar spikes and other health concerns.

Non-Compliance with Reverse Type 2 Diabetes Diet: Such foods typically conflict with the principles of the Reverse Type 2 Diabetes Diet and the 2020-2025 Dietary Guidelines for Americans.

The breading used in these dishes is often high in carbohydrates and can lead to unexpected spikes in blood sugar levels. Additionally, these foods are typically deep-fried, a process that significantly increases their fat and calorie content, potentially leading to weight gain - a risk factor for T2D.

In addition, it is important to note that the frying process can contribute to the production of Advanced Glycation End-products (AGEs). AGEs are compounds that form when proteins or fats in the bloodstream react with sugar, and have been associated with aging as well as chronic or degenerative diseases, such as chronic kidney disease, atherosclerosis, and diabetes.

These meals also commonly lack adequate dietary fiber, an essential nutrient for managing blood sugar levels and promoting overall digestive health.

Due to their high levels of carbohydrates and fats, low fiber content, and the potential formation of AGEs, breaded and fried foods are generally discouraged for individuals managing or aiming to reverse type 2 diabetes (T2D). When following a Reverse Type 2 Diabetes Diet, it is crucial to make informed food choices, prioritize fresh and minimally processed options, and restrict the consumption of fried and breaded foods.

Ⓢ *Chicken fingers* Ⓢ *Chicken fried steak* Ⓢ *Chicken nuggets* Ⓢ *Chicken Parmesan* Ⓢ *Chicken tenders/strips* Ⓢ *Fish and chips* Ⓢ *Fried alligator* Ⓢ *Fried apple fritters* Ⓢ *Fried artichoke hearts* Ⓢ *Fried avocado slices* Ⓢ *Fried bacon* Ⓢ *Fried baloney sandwich* Ⓢ *Fried bologna* Ⓢ *Fried calamari* Ⓢ *Fried catfish* Ⓢ *Fried cheese sticks* Ⓢ *Fried cheeseburgers* Ⓢ *Fried chicken and waffles* Ⓢ *Fried chicken breast* Ⓢ *Fried chicken drumsticks* Ⓢ *Fried chicken sandwich* Ⓢ *Fried chicken thighs* Ⓢ *Fried chicken wings* Ⓢ *Fried cinnamon sugar doughnuts* Ⓢ *Fried clams* Ⓢ *Fried corn nuggets* Ⓢ *Fried crab cake sandwich* Ⓢ *Fried crab cakes* Ⓢ *Fried crawfish* Ⓢ *Fried dumplings* Ⓢ *Fried egg rolls* Ⓢ *Fried empanadas* Ⓢ *Fried fish sandwich* Ⓢ *Fried French toast sticks* Ⓢ *Fried frog legs* Ⓢ *Fried green beans* Ⓢ *Fried green tomatoes* Ⓢ *Fried ham* Ⓢ *Fried hot dogs* Ⓢ *Fried ice cream* Ⓢ *Fried jalapeno poppers* Ⓢ *Fried liver* Ⓢ *Fried lobster* Ⓢ *Fried lobster roll* Ⓢ *Fried mac and cheese bites* Ⓢ *Fried meatball sandwich* Ⓢ *Fried mozzarella bites* Ⓢ *Fried mushrooms* Ⓢ *Fried okra* Ⓢ *Fried onion rings* Ⓢ *Fried Oreos* Ⓢ *Fried oysters* Ⓢ *Fried PB&J sandwich* Ⓢ *Fried pickles* Ⓢ *Fried plantains* Ⓢ *Fried polenta sticks* Ⓢ *Fried pork chops* Ⓢ *Fried pork ribs* Ⓢ *Fried samosas* Ⓢ *Fried sausage links/patties* Ⓢ *Fried scallops* Ⓢ *Fried shrimp* Ⓢ *Fried shrimp po' boy sandwich* Ⓢ *Fried spring rolls* Ⓢ *Fried steak sandwich* Ⓢ *Fried sweet potato fries* Ⓢ *Fried tofu* Ⓢ

Fried turkey legs ⊘ *Fried wontons* ⊘ *Fried zucchini sticks*

HIGH-CARB BREAKFAST ITEMS

High-Carb Breakfast Items like pancakes, waffles, French toast, and sweetened cereals are common choices in American restaurants. While they might be popular, these dishes are laden with carbohydrates that can cause significant spikes in blood sugar levels, making them incompatible with a Type 2 Diabetes (T2D) reversal diet.

Non-Compliance with Reverse Type 2 Diabetes Diet: High-carb breakfast items often conflict with the principles of the Reverse Type 2 Diabetes Diet and the Dietary Guidelines for Americans. Loaded with carbohydrates, these dishes can cause sharp rises in blood sugar levels, posing challenges to blood sugar control and weight management.

These breakfast options are typically made from refined grains, lacking the fiber found in whole grains. Dietary fiber is crucial in regulating blood sugar levels, as it decelerates the absorption of sugar into the bloodstream, thereby preventing rapid spikes in blood sugar. The lack of fiber in these foods allows for quicker absorption of sugars, leading to more rapid increases in blood glucose levels.

Furthermore, these items can be served in large portions and may be topped with sweet syrups or fruit compotes, adding to their overall sugar and calorie content. This can contribute to weight gain, a major risk factor for T2D.

When it comes to managing or reversing T2D, it's important to make mindful choices about what to eat, especially at the start of the day. Opting for high-protein, low-carbohydrate options, or whole grains can help better manage blood sugar levels and support overall health. As such, high-carb breakfast items like pancakes, waffles, and sweetened cereals are generally not recommended for those following a Reverse Type 2 Diabetes Diet.

LARGE BURGERS

These often contain multiple patties, layers of cheese, bacon, and sweet sauces, making them calorie-dense and potentially contributing to weight gain, which is not beneficial for individuals following a Type 2 Diabetes (T2D) reversal diet.

Non-Compliance with Reverse Type 2 Diabetes Diet: Large, loaded burgers typically do not align with the principles of the Reverse Type 2 Diabetes Diet or the 2020-2025 Dietary Guidelines for Americans.

The components of these burgers - particularly the large meat patties and toppings like cheese and bacon - can contribute significantly to the meal's overall fat and calorie content. Consuming such high-calorie meals can make it challenging to maintain a healthy weight, a crucial aspect of managing and reversing T2D.

Additionally, the sweet sauces often added to these burgers can contain high amounts of added sugars, leading to unexpected spikes in blood glucose levels. The buns used for these burgers are also typically made from refined grains, which are high in carbohydrates and have a high glycemic index, potentially leading to further blood sugar spikes.

Moreover, large burgers often lack balance in terms of nutrients. They are generally low in fiber, a key nutrient for regulating blood glucose levels, and can also be high in sodium, contributing to elevated blood pressure, a common concern for individuals with diabetes.

Due to their high calorie, fat, and sodium content, as well as their potential to cause blood sugar spikes, it is generally advised for individuals managing or reversing type 2 diabetes (T2D) to avoid consuming large, loaded burgers. Making mindful choices, such as selecting leaner meats, incorporating vegetables, and opting for whole-grain buns, can help make burgers a healthier option.

However, it is crucial to maintain portion control when enjoying a burger.

⊘ *Bacon avocado burger* ⊘ *Bacon cheeseburger* ⊘ *BBQ bacon cheeseburger* ⊘ *BBQ pulled pork burger* ⊘ *BBQ ranch burger* ⊘ *BLT burger with bacon, lettuce, and tomato* ⊘ *Blue cheeseburger* ⊘ *Breakfast burger with bacon, egg, and cheese* ⊘ *Breakfast sausage burger with egg and cheese* ⊘ *Brunch burger with fried egg, bacon, and hash browns* ⊘ *Buffalo chicken burger with hot sauce and blue cheese dressing* ⊘ *Cajun blackened burger with spicy seasoning* ⊘ *Caprese burger with mozzarella, tomato, and basil* ⊘ *Chili cheeseburger* ⊘ *Chili dog burger with chili and hot dog slices* ⊘ *Double cheeseburger* ⊘ *Fajita burger with grilled peppers and onions* ⊘ *Fried egg burger* ⊘ *Fried onion burger with crispy fried onions* ⊘ *Garlic mushroom burger* ⊘ *Gourmet blue cheese and fig burger* ⊘ *Gourmet burger with foie gras and truffle aioli* ⊘ *Greek lamb burger with feta cheese and tzatziki sauce* ⊘ *Guacamole bacon burger* ⊘ *Guacamole ranch burger* ⊘ *Hawaiian BBQ burger with BBQ sauce, pineapple, and ham* ⊘ *Hawaiian burger with grilled pineapple and ham* ⊘ *Italian burger with marinara sauce and melted cheese* ⊘ *Jalapeno popper burger* ⊘ *Mac and cheese burger* ⊘ *Mexican burger with salsa, guacamole, and jalapenos* ⊘ *Mushroom Swiss burger* ⊘ *Nacho burger with tortilla chips, cheese, and salsa* ⊘ *Pastrami burger with sliced pastrami and mustard* ⊘ *Patty melt with Swiss cheese and grilled onions* ⊘ *Peanut butter bacon burger* ⊘ *Philly cheesesteak burger* ⊘ *Pimento cheeseburger* ⊘ *Pretzel bun burger* ⊘ *Prime rib burger* ⊘ *Reuben burger with sauerkraut and Thousand Island dressing* ⊘ *Smoked Gouda burger* ⊘ *Southwest burger with spicy sauce,*

jalapenos, and avocado ⊘ *Sriracha bacon burger* ⊘
Stuffed burger with cheese or other fillings ⊘ *Teriyaki*
bacon burger ⊘ *Teriyaki pineapple burger* ⊘ *Triple*
cheeseburger ⊘ *Turkey burger with cranberry sauce and*
stuffing ⊘ *Veggie burger with cheese and avocado*

SWEETENED DESSERTS

Foods like cakes, pies, cookies, and ice cream are typically laden with added sugars, unhealthy fats, and refined carbohydrates, all of which can pose challenges for individuals following a Type 2 Diabetes (T2D) reversal diet.

Non-Compliance with Reverse Type 2 Diabetes Diet: These dessert items often do not align with the principles of the Reverse Type 2 Diabetes Diet or the 2020-2025 Dietary Guidelines for Americans.

Sweetened desserts are typically high in added sugars, which can cause rapid spikes in blood glucose levels, contributing to unstable blood sugar control. These foods can also be high in unhealthy fats, particularly trans fats and saturated fats, which can increase the risk of heart disease, a common concern for individuals with diabetes.

Moreover, a significant number of these desserts are prepared using refined grains that are deficient in fiber, resulting in potential blood sugar spikes. The absence of fiber in these foods also contributes to a high glycemic index, which further intensifies blood sugar spikes and extends periods of elevated blood sugar levels.

Additionally, the high calorie content found in sweetened desserts can contribute to weight gain, further compounding the difficulties of managing and reversing type 2 diabetes (T2D).

Considering their high levels of sugar, fat, and calories, as well as their capacity to induce substantial blood sugar spikes, it is advised to avoid sweetened desserts when managing or reversing type 2 diabetes

(T2D). Instead, if a craving for something sweet arises, it is advisable to opt for fresh fruits or desserts prepared with sugar substitutes, while also remaining conscious of portion sizes.

Apple pie ⊘ *Baklava* ⊘ *Banana split* ⊘ *Bread pudding* ⊘ *Brownies* ⊘ *Cannoli* ⊘ *Caramel apples* ⊘ *Carrot cake* ⊘ *Cheesecake* ⊘ *Chocolate cake* ⊘ *Chocolate chip cookies* ⊘ *Chocolate fondue* ⊘ *Chocolate mousse* ⊘ *Chocolate-covered strawberries* ⊘ *Churros* ⊘ *Cinnamon rolls* ⊘ *Coconut macaroons* ⊘ *Crème brûlée* ⊘ *Danish pastries* ⊘ *Donuts* ⊘ *Éclair* ⊘ *Flan* ⊘ *Fried dough or funnel cake* ⊘ *Fruit cobbler* ⊘ *Fruit crumble* ⊘ *Fruit tart* ⊘ *Fruit-filled turnovers* ⊘ *Fudge* ⊘ *Ice cream cones with sugary toppings* ⊘ *Ice cream sundaes* ⊘ *Key lime pie* ⊘ *Lemon bars* ⊘ *Macarons* ⊘ *Marshmallow treats* ⊘ *Milkshakes* ⊘ *Muffins with added sugars* ⊘ *Oatmeal raisin cookies* ⊘ *Panna cotta* ⊘ *Peanut butter cookies* ⊘ *Pecan pie* ⊘ *Popsicles with added sugars* ⊘ *Pumpkin pie* ⊘ *Red velvet cake* ⊘ *Rice pudding* ⊘ *S'mores* ⊘ *Strawberry shortcake* ⊘ *Sugar cookies* ⊘ *Sweet crepes* ⊘ *Tiramisu* ⊘ *Vanilla cake*

CREAMY AND HIGH-FAT SALAD DRESSINGS

Creamy and High-Fat Salad Dressings: Salad dressings, particularly creamy varieties like ranch or Caesar, can be high in unhealthy fats and calories. While they may seem like a simple addition to a salad, their potential impact on blood sugar levels and overall health can be substantial.

Non-Compliance with Reverse Type 2 Diabetes Diet: These types of salad dressings often do not align with the principles of the Reverse Type 2 Diabetes Diet or the 2020-2025 Dietary Guidelines for Americans.

Creamy and high-fat salad dressings often contain significant amounts of saturated fats, which can raise cholesterol levels and heighten the likelihood of heart disease. This becomes particularly concerning for individuals with type 2 diabetes (T2D), as they already face an elevated risk of cardiovascular complications.

Furthermore, these dressings can be high in calories, contributing to excess caloric intake and potential weight gain. Weight management is a critical component of the T2D reversal process, and the high-calorie content of these dressings can pose a challenge to maintaining or achieving a healthy weight.

Additionally, many commercially prepared salad dressings also contain added sugars, which can lead to unexpected blood sugar spikes. They may also contain preservatives and other additives that can interfere with overall health.

Considering their high levels of unhealthy fats, calories, and potential sugar content, it is advisable for individuals managing or reversing type 2 diabetes (T2D) to avoid creamy and high-fat salad dressings. Healthier alternatives such as vinaigrettes, lemon juice, or a small amount of olive oil can be chosen instead, as they are lower in saturated fats and sugars. Additionally, when using salad dressing, it is recommended to have it on the side to have better control over the portion size.

Avocado ranch dressing ⊘ *Blue cheese dressing* ⊘ *Buttermilk dressing* ⊘ *Caesar dressing* ⊘ *Chipotle ranch dressing* ⊘ *Creamy almond dressing* ⊘ *Creamy avocado dressing* ⊘ *Creamy bacon dressing* ⊘ *Creamy balsamic dressing* ⊘ *Creamy blue cheese dressing* ⊘ *Creamy Caesar dressing* ⊘ *Creamy cashew dressing* ⊘ *Creamy chipotle dressing* ⊘ *Creamy cilantro lime dressing* ⊘ *Creamy coconut dressing* ⊘ *Creamy cucumber dressing* ⊘ *Creamy curry dressing* ⊘ *Creamy dill dressing* ⊘

Creamy French dressing Ⓢ *Creamy garlic dressing* Ⓢ
Creamy ginger dressing Ⓢ *Creamy ginger miso dressing*
Ⓢ *Creamy honey mustard dressing* Ⓢ *Creamy*
horseradish dressing Ⓢ *Creamy Italian dressing* Ⓢ
Creamy Italian herb dressing Ⓢ *Creamy lemon herb*
dressing Ⓢ *Creamy macadamia nut dressing* Ⓢ *Creamy*
mango dressing Ⓢ *Creamy maple dijon dressing* Ⓢ
Creamy Parmesan dressing Ⓢ *Creamy peanut dressing*
Ⓢ *Creamy pecan dressing* Ⓢ *Creamy pesto dressing* Ⓢ
Creamy pineapple dressing Ⓢ *Creamy ranch dressing* Ⓢ
Creamy roasted garlic dressing Ⓢ *Creamy Russian*
dressing Ⓢ *Creamy sesame dressing* Ⓢ *Creamy sesame*
ginger dressing Ⓢ *Creamy sriracha dressing* Ⓢ *Creamy*
sun-dried tomato dressing Ⓢ *Creamy sunflower seed*
dressing Ⓢ *Creamy sweet chili dressing* Ⓢ *Creamy tahini*
dressing Ⓢ *Creamy walnut dressing* Ⓢ *Green goddess*
dressing Ⓢ *Honey mustard dressing (creamy variety)* Ⓢ
Ranch dressing Ⓢ *Thousand Island dressing*

* * *

In the subsequent section of this chapter, comprehensive tables are provided to outline foods that are non-compliant with Reverse Type 2 Diabetes Diet. These tables offer detailed information including serving size, Glycemic Index (GI), Glycemic Load (GL), and Net Carbohydrates for each food item. These metrics are particularly relevant when a food item's non-compliance is attributed to a high glycemic load and/or high carbohydrate content.

However, it is important to note that not all non-compliant foods can be categorized solely based on their GI, GL, or net carbohydrate content. Some food items are deemed non-compliant due to factors such as extensive processing, excessive sodium content, or an abundance of unhealthy fats. For these specific food items, detailed GI, GL, or net carb data may not be provided in the tables. Instead, they are simply listed with a note indicating their non-compliant status. This differentiation is aimed at ensuring clarity in understanding why certain food items are not recommended under the principles of the Reverse Type 2 Diabetes Diet.

AMERICAN RESTAURANT FOODS

AMERICAN RESTAURANT FOOD	SERVING SIZE	GI	GL	NET CARB
Apple Pie	½ slice (62g)	55	11	20g
Bacon Cheese Fries	1 cup (156g)	70	31.5	45g
Bagel, plain	1 medium (105g)	70	33.6	48g
BBQ Pulled Pork Sandwich	1 sandwich (200g)	55	22	40g
Beef Burrito	1 burrito (200g)	55	24.8	45g
Biscuits and Gravy	1 serving (256g)	70	26.6	38g
BLT Sandwich	1 sandwich (219g)	50	18	36g
Buffalo Chicken Wrap	1 wrap (210g)	60	21	35g
Cheese Fries	1 serving	Non-compliant Foods		
Cheese Quesadilla	1 quesadilla (170g)	50	12.5	25g
Cheeseburger	1 burger (200g)	60	19.2	32g
Chicken Alfredo Pasta	1.5 cups (200g)	50	20	40g
Chicken and Biscuits	1 serving	Non-compliant Foods		
Chicken and Broccoli Alfredo	1.5 cups (200g)	50	22.5	45g
Chicken and Dumplings	1 serving (300g)	55	19.3	35g
Chicken and Waffles	1 serving (200g)	60	30	50g
Chicken Fried Rice	1.5 cups (246g)	60	28.8	48g
Chicken Fried Steak	1 serving	Non-compliant Foods		
Chicken Lo Mein	1.5 cups (246g)	55	27.5	50g
Chicken Parmesan	1 piece (174g)	60	24	40g
Chicken Pot Pie	1 piece (200g)	60	24	40g
Chicken Quesadilla	1 quesadilla (200g)	65	23.4	36g

AMERICAN RESTAURANT FOOD	SERVING SIZE	GI	GL	NET CARB
Chili Cheese Dog	1 serving	Non-compliant Foods		
Chili Cheese Fries	1 serving (200g)	75	37.5	50g
Clam Chowder	1 cup (240g)	55	11	20g
Clam Strips	1 serving (180g)	60	15	25g
Club Sandwich	1 sandwich (233g)	50	17.5	35g
Corn Dog	1 corn dog (110g)	60	15	25g
Deep Dish Pizza	1 serving	Non-compliant Foods		
Eggs Benedict	1 serving (242g)	50	15	30g
Eggs Benedict with Hash Browns	1 serving	Non-compliant Foods		
Enchiladas	1 serving	Non-compliant Foods		
Fish and Chips	1 serving (284g)	70	46.9	67g
French Fries	1 serving (100g)	75	26.3	35g
Fried Calamari	1 serving	Non-compliant Foods		
Fried Catfish	1 fillet (200g)	Non-compliant Foods		
Fried Chicken	2 pieces (150g)	50	10	20g
Fried Chicken and Waffles	1 serving	Non-compliant Foods		
Fried Chicken Sandwich	1 serving	Non-compliant Foods		
Fried Green Tomatoes	1 serving (150g)	55	11	20g
Fried Shrimp	6 pieces (126g)	60	13.2	22g
Grilled Cheese	1 sandwich (134g)	60	18	30g
Gumbo, shrimp	1 serving (300g)	50	10	20g
Hot Dog with Bun	1 hot dog (150g)	60	18	30g
Loaded Nachos	1 serving	Non-compliant Foods		
Lobster Mac and Cheese	1 cup (200g)	60	27	45g
Lobster Roll	1 roll (220g)	50	20	40g
Macaroni and Cheese	1 serving (200g)	65	26	40g

AMERICAN RESTAURANT FOOD	SERVING SIZE	GI	GL	NET CARB
Meatball Sub	1 sub (300g)	55	19.3	35g
Mozzarella Sticks	6 sticks (180g)	55	19.3	35g
Nachos with Cheese	1 serving (180g)	70	21	30g
Onion Rings	8-9 rings (83g)	60	21	35g
Onion Soup	1 cup (240g)	55	11	20g
Pancakes with Syrup	2 pancakes (232g)	70	31.5	45g
Peanut Butter and Jelly Sandwich	1 sandwich (150g)	55	19.3	35g
Pecan Pie	1 slice (150g)	50	20	40g
Philly Cheese Steak	1 sandwich (269g)	60	25.2	42g
Philly Cheesesteak	1 serving	Non-compliant Foods		
Pizza, pepperoni	2 slices (128g)	60	21.6	36g
Pot Pie (Chicken or Beef)	1 serving	Non-compliant Foods		
Pulled Chicken Sandwich	1 sandwich (200g)	55	11	20g
Red Velvet Cake	1 slice (150g)	55	27.5	50g
Reuben Sandwich	1 sandwich (233g)	60	21.6	36g
Roast Beef Sandwich	1 sandwich (200g)	50	12.5	25g
S'mores	1 serving (100g)	70	21	30g
Sausage, Egg and Cheese Biscuit	1 biscuit (174g)	55	17.6	32g
Shrimp and Grits	1 serving (250g)	45	13.5	30g
Sloppy Joe	1 sandwich (250g)	60	21	35g
Spaghetti and Meatballs	1 serving (300g)	55	24.8	45g
Steak Fajitas	2 fajitas (200g)	55	17.6	32g
Stuffed Crust Pizza	1 serving	Non-compliant Foods		
Sweet Potato Casserole	1 cup (200g)	70	35	50g

AMERICAN RESTAURANT FOOD	SERVING SIZE	GI	GL	NET CARB
Tacos	2 tacos (200g)	60	21	35g
Tomato Soup with Grilled Cheese	1 serving (350g)	55	27.5	50g
Tuna Salad Sandwich	1 sandwich (219g)	50	20	40g
Turkey Club Sandwich	1 sandwich (200g)	45	13.5	30g
Veggie Burger	1 burger (200g)	40	10	25g
White Chocolate Raspberry Cheesecake	1 slice (150g)	60	24	40g
Wild Rice Pilaf	1 serving (200g)	50	17.5	35g
Zucchini Bread	1 slice (80g)	60	12	20g
Sweet Potato Casserole	1 cup (200g)	70	35	50g
Tacos	2 tacos (200g)	60	21	35g
Tomato Soup with Grilled Cheese	1 serving (350g)	55	27.5	50g
Tuna Salad Sandwich	1 sandwich (219g)	50	20	40g
Turkey Club Sandwich	1 sandwich (200g)	45	13.5	30g
Veggie Burger	1 burger (200g)	40	10	25g
White Chocolate Raspberry Cheesecake	1 slice (150g)	60	24	40g
Wild Rice Pilaf	1 serving (200g)	50	17.5	35g
Zucchini Bread	1 slice (80g)	60	12	20g

BREADS AND BAKED PRODUCTS

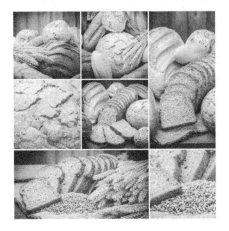

Bread and baked products that do not align with the principles of a Type 2 Diabetes (T2D) reversal diet include:

- **White Bread**: White bread is derived from refined grains that undergo a process where their fiber and nutrient content is depleted. As a result, it possesses a high glycemic index, leading to rapid and significant elevations in blood sugar levels.

- **Sweetened or flavored breads:** Breads with added sugars, such as cinnamon raisin bread, sweet fruit breads, or sweet rolls, can significantly increase carbohydrate and sugar intake, leading to elevated blood sugar levels.
- **Pastries and sweet baked goods**: Pastries, including croissants, doughnuts, muffins, and sweet rolls, are often made with high amounts of butter, sugar, and refined flour, making them calorie-dense and rich in carbohydrates.
- **Sweet Breads and Rolls**: These include products like cinnamon rolls and danishes, which are high in sugar and low in fiber.
- **Bagels**: A single bagel can contain the equivalent amount of carbohydrates as several slices of bread, leading to potential blood sugar spikes.
- **Biscuits and Scones**: These tend to be high in unhealthy fats and low in fiber, making them less suitable for a Reverse Type 2 Diabetes Diet.
- **Flavored and Sweetened Cornbread**: Traditional cornbread may not be as problematic, but varieties that include sweeteners can be high in sugar and less suitable for a Reverse Type 2 Diabetes Diet.
- **Sugary muffins and cakes:** Muffins, cupcakes, cakes, and cake-like desserts made with refined flour, added sugars, and high-fat ingredients can be detrimental to blood sugar control and weight management.
- **Sugar-laden cookies and pastries:** Cookies, pastries, and baked goods made with refined flour and large amounts of added sugars can lead to blood sugar imbalances and contribute to excess calorie intake.
- **High-carb crackers and pretzels:** Crackers and pretzels made from refined grains are typically high in carbohydrates and lack fiber, causing rapid increases in blood sugar levels.

* * *

In the subsequent section of this chapter, comprehensive tables are provided to outline foods that are non-compliant with Reverse Type 2 Diabetes Diet. These tables offer detailed information including serving size, Glycemic Index (GI), Glycemic Load (GL), and Net Carbohydrates for each food item. These metrics are particularly relevant when a food item's non-compliance is attributed to a high glycemic load and/or high carbohydrate content.

However, it is important to note that not all non-compliant foods can be categorized solely based on their GI, GL, or net carbohydrate content. Some food items are deemed non-compliant due to factors such as extensive processing, excessive sodium content, or an abundance of unhealthy fats. For these specific food items, detailed GI, GL, or net carb data may not be provided in the tables. Instead, they are simply listed with a note indicating their non-compliant status. This differentiation is aimed at ensuring clarity in understanding why certain food items are not recommended under the principles of the Reverse Type 2 Diabetes Diet.

BREADS AND BAKED PRODUCTS

FRUITS & FRUIT PRODUCTS	SERVING SIZE	GI	GL	NET CARB
MEDIUM GLYCEMIC LOAD FOODS (Eat occasionally, and reduce the serving size to stay below 15 grams of net carbs)				
Apple Pie	1 slice, 125g	40	18	32g
Apple Turnover	1 medium, 100g	45	15	33g
Bacon Cheddar Biscuits	1 biscuit, 64g	62	12	25g
Bakewell Tart	1 slice, 80g	45	16	35g
Baklava	1 piece, 33g	51	15	29g
Bannock	1 piece, 60g	70	12	24g
Beignets	1 medium, 60g	50	17	34g
Biscuit Sandwiches	1 sandwich, 130g	62	12	28g
Black Forest Cake	1 slice, 100g	35	12	34g
Black Forest Tart	1 slice, 100g	65	16	25g
Blackberry Pie	1 slice, 125g	55	15	29g
Blueberry Custard Tart	1 slice, 100g	55	14	21g
Blueberry Pie	1 slice, 125g	60	17	30g
Boston Cream Pie	1 slice, 100g	35	12	34g
Buttermilk Biscuits	1 biscuit, 64g	62	11	24g
Buttermilk Pie	1 slice, 125g	50	17	38g
Cannoli	1 medium, 85g	50	16	32g
Carrot Cake	1 slice, 100g	40	16	40g
Challah	1 slice, 40g	60	12	20g
Cheesecake	1 slice, 100g	35	10	28g
Chocolate Cake	1 slice, 100g	38	14	35g
Chocolate Chip Biscuits	1 biscuit, 57g	62	14	33g

FRUITS & FRUIT PRODUCTS	SERVING SIZE	GI	GL	NET CARB
Chocolate Chip Cookies	1 cookie, 30g	65	11	19g
Chocolate Silk Pie	1 slice, 100g	65	19	26g
Chocolate Tart	1 slice, 100g	70	10	23g
Churros	1 medium, 30g	45	11	24g
Ciabatta	1 serving, 50g	65	12	20g
Cinnamon Roll	1 small, 60g	50	16	31g
Cinnamon Roll Biscuits	1 biscuit, 28g	65	10	20g
Coconut Cake	1 slice, 80g	70	18	31g
Coconut Cream Pie	1 slice, 100g	60	16	26g
Coffee Cake	1 slice, 100g	37	14	38g
Cornbread	1 piece, 60g	65	18	28g
Cornish Pasty	1 small, 150g	45	18	40g
Croissant	1 medium,57g	47	12	23g
Custard Tart	1 slice, 100g	60	10	20g
Dobos Torte	1 slice, 100g	35	11	31g
Double Chocolate Cookies	1 cookie, 30g	70	13	19g
Eccles Cake	1 cake, 60g	50	13	27g
Éclair	1 medium, 85g	46	12	26g
Empanada	1 small, 100g	40	14	35g
Focaccia	1 slice, 50g	65	12	20g
Fougasse	1 serving, 50g	65	12	20g
French Bread	1 slice, 30g	95	14	15g
German Chocolate Cake	1 slice, 100g	38	15	38g
Gingerbread Cookies	1 cookie, 30g	65	10	16g
Ham and Cheese Biscuits	1 biscuit, 60g	62	10	20g
Irish Soda Bread	1 slice, 45g	65	13	20g
Italian Bread	1 slice, 30g	70	10	14g
Lemon Cake	1 slice, 100g	34	11	31g

FRUITS & FRUIT PRODUCTS	SERVING SIZE	GI	GL	NET CARB
Lemon Meringue Pie	1 slice, 125g	45	17	31g
Lemon Mousse Tart	1 slice, 100g	45	11	22g
Linzer Cookies	1 cookie, 30g	55	10	16g
M&M Cookies	1 cookie, 30g	65	11	19g
Marble Cake	1 slice, 100g	34	13	36g
Mille Crepe Cake	1 slice, 100g	30	10	33g
Mixed Berry Pie	1 slice, 100g	65	14	18g
Molasses Cookies	1 cookie, 30g	60	12	17g
Naan	1 piece, 60g	62	16	26g
Oatmeal Raisin Cookies	1 cookie, 30g	55	10	16g
Orange Cake	1 slice, 80g	70	18	31g
Panettone	1 slice, 50g	65	15	23g
Peach Pie	1 slice, 125g	50	16	27g
Pita Bread	1 small pita, 35g	57	10	18g
Pithivier	1 small, 90g	50	18	36g
Pound Cake	1 slice, 100g	34	13	37g
Pretzel	1 medium, 60g	75	16	22g
Puff Pastry	1 sheet, 79g	50	18	36g
Rhubarb Pie	1 slice, 125g	50	14	26g
Simit	1 piece, 60g	65	14	22g
Sponge Cake	1 slice, 100g	32	11	33g
Strawberry Shortcake	1 slice, 100g	34	11	32g
Strawberry Tart	1 biscuit, 50g	62	10	22g
Sugar Cookies	1 slice, 100g	45	17	38g
Sweet Potato Biscuits	1 cookie, 30g	65	10	16g
Tiramisu	1 small, 60g	45	13	28g
Tomato Tart	1 slice, 100g	40	12	30g
Vol-au-vent	1 slice, 100g	36	13	34g

FRUITS & FRUIT PRODUCTS	SERVING SIZE	GI	GL	NET CARB
Molasses Cookies	1 cookie, 30g	60	12	17g
Naan	1 piece, 60g	62	16	26g
Oatmeal Raisin Cookies	1 cookie, 30g	55	10	16g
Orange Cake	1 slice, 80g	70	18	31g
Panettone	1 slice, 50g	65	15	23g
Peach Pie	1 slice, 125g	50	16	27g
Pita Bread	1 small pita, 35g	57	10	18g
Pithivier	1 small, 90g	50	18	36g
Pound Cake	1 slice, 100g	34	13	37g
Pretzel	1 medium, 60g	75	16	22g
Puff Pastry	1 sheet, 79g	50	18	36g
Rhubarb Pie	1 slice, 125g	50	14	26g
Simit	1 piece, 60g	65	14	22g
Sponge Cake	1 slice, 100g	32	11	33g
Strawberry Shortcake	1 slice, 100g	34	11	32g
Strawberry Tart	1 biscuit, 50g	62	10	22g
Sugar Cookies	1 slice, 100g	45	17	38g
Sweet Potato Biscuits	1 cookie, 30g	65	10	16g
Tiramisu	1 small, 60g	45	13	28g
Tomato Tart	1 slice, 100g	40	12	30g
Vol-au-vent	1 slice, 100g	36	13	34g
HIGH GLYCEMIC LOAD FOODS				
Baguette	1 serving, 50g	95	23	25g
Almond Poppy Seed Bread (store bought)	1 serving, 50g	High	High	Varies
Apple Cinnamon Muffins (store bought)	1 serving, 50g	High	High	Varies
Banana Bread (store bought)	1 serving, 50g	High	High	Varies

FRUITS & FRUIT PRODUCTS	SERVING SIZE	GI	GL	NET CARB
Blueberry Muffins (store bought)	1 serving, 50g	High	High	Varies
Carrot Muffins (store bought)	1 serving, 50g	High	High	Varies
Cherry Pie	1 slice, 125g	70	21	31g
Chocolate Chip Muffins (store bought)	1 serving, 50g	High	High	Varies
Chocolate Pecan Pie	1 slice, 125g	55	23.1	42g
Cinnamon Swirl Bread (store bought)	1 serving, 50g	High	High	Varies
Coffee Cake (store bought)	1 serving, 50g	High	High	Varies
Commercially-prepared cakes with added frosting, fillings, or glazes.	1 serving, 50g	High	High	Varies
commercially-prepared cookies with added frosting, fillings, or glazes.	1 serving, 50g	High	High	Varies
Commercially-prepared cupcakes with added frosting, fillings, or glazes.	1 serving, 50g	High	High	Varies
Cranberry Orange Bread (store bought)	1 serving, 50g	High	High	Varies
Danish Pastry	1 medium, 84g	59	22	37g
Double Chocolate Muffins (store bought)	1 serving, 50g	High	High	Varies
Hummingbird Cake	1 slice, 80g	67	21	37g
Key Lime Pie	1 serving, 50g	High	High	Varies
Lemon Meringue Pie	1 serving, 50g	High	High	Varies
Lemon Poppy Seed Muffins (store bought)	1 serving, 50g	High	High	Varies
Mississippi Mud Pie	1 slice, 100g	60	24	30g
Opera Cake	1 slice, 80g	65	23	28g

FRUITS & FRUIT PRODUCTS	SERVING SIZE	GI	GL	NET CARB
Peach Muffins (store bought)	1 serving, 50g	High	High	Varies
Pecan Pie	1 slice, 125g	50	26	41g
Pretzels (store bought)	1 serving, 50g	High	High	Varies
Pumpkin Bread (store bought)	1 serving, 50g	High	High	Varies
Pumpkin Pie	1 slice, 125g	75	22	30g
Raspberry Streusel Bread (store bought)	1 serving, 50g	High	High	Varies
Rice Cakes	1 serving, 50g	High	High	Varies
Vanilla Cake	1 slice, 100g	65	22	42g
Waffles with sugary syrups	1 serving, 50g	High	High	Varies
Zucchini Bread (store bought)	1 serving, 50g	High	High	Varies

LEGUMES AND PULSES

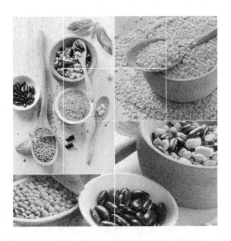

While legumes and pulses are generally good for people with type 2 diabetes because they are high in fiber and can help regulate blood sugar, there are a few cases where they might not align with a Reverse Type 2 Diabetes Diet:

CANNED BEANS

Often, these are high in added sugars and sodium. It's best to opt for low-sodium, low-sugar varieties or make your own at home.

REFRIED BEANS

When referring to specific brands or types of refried beans not suitable for a Type 2 Diabetes (T2D) reversal diet, the main concern is usually about added unhealthy fats, high sodium content, or potentially added sugars. Here are some general categories of refried beans that are not compliant with Reverse Type 2 Diabetes Diet:

Canned Refried Beans with Added Fats: Some refried beans are cooked with added fats, often unhealthy ones, which can contribute to calorie overload and weight gain.

Canned Refried Beans with High Sodium: Sodium is often added for flavor and preservation. Excessive sodium can contribute to high blood pressure, a common comorbidity with T2D.

Canned Refried Beans with Added Sugars: While not as common, some brands may add sugars to their refried beans, which can contribute to elevated blood glucose levels.

Restaurant-Served Refried Beans: Restaurants may prepare their refried beans with substantial amounts of unhealthy fats or add ingredients high in sodium or sugar.

Refried Beans with Full-Fat Cheese: Refried beans are often served with cheese. Full-fat cheese can contribute to calorie and saturated fat intake.

Flavored Refried Beans: Some versions of refried beans come with additional flavorings or ingredients, which can add to their sugar, fat, and sodium content.

Black Bean Refried Beans ◊ Cheesy Refried Beans ◊

Creamy Refried Beans Ⓢ *Cuban-Style Refried Beans* Ⓢ
Frijoles Charros (Refried Beans with Bacon and Chorizo)
Ⓢ *Green Chile Refried Beans* Ⓢ *Guajillo Refried Beans*
Ⓢ *Instant Pot Refried Beans* Ⓢ *Jalapeño Refried Beans*
Ⓢ *Mexican-Style Refried Beans* Ⓢ *Pinto Bean Refried*
Beans Ⓢ *Ranch-Style Refried Beans* Ⓢ *Refried Beans*
with Avocado Ⓢ *Refried Beans with Bacon* Ⓢ *Refried*
Beans with Caramelized Onions Ⓢ *Refried Beans with*
Cheddar Cheese Ⓢ *Refried Beans with Cheese* Ⓢ *Refried*
Beans with Chipotle Powder Ⓢ *Refried Beans with*
Chorizo Ⓢ *Refried Beans with Cilantro* Ⓢ *Refried Beans*
with Corn Ⓢ *Refried Beans with Cumin* Ⓢ *Refried*
Beans with Epazote Ⓢ *Refried Beans with Epazote and*
Cumin Ⓢ *Refried Beans with Garlic* Ⓢ *Refried Beans*
with Green Onions Ⓢ *Refried Beans with Ground Beef*
Ⓢ *Refried Beans with Guacamole* Ⓢ *Refried Beans with*
Guajillo Chili Powder Ⓢ *Refried Beans with Jalapeños* Ⓢ
Refried Beans with Lime Ⓢ *Refried Beans with Mexican*
Crema Ⓢ *Refried Beans with Onion* Ⓢ *Refried Beans*
with Oregano Ⓢ *Refried Beans with Paprika* Ⓢ *Refried*
Beans with Pico de Gallo Ⓢ *Refried Beans with Queso*
Fresco Ⓢ *Refried Beans with Red Pepper Flakes* Ⓢ
Refried Beans with Salsa Ⓢ *Refried Beans with Serrano*
Peppers Ⓢ *Refried Beans with Smoked Paprika* Ⓢ
Refried Beans with Sour Cream Ⓢ *Refried Beans with*
Tomatoes Ⓢ *Refried Black Beans with Cilantro* Ⓢ *Slow*
Cooker Refried Beans Ⓢ *Smoky Chipotle Refried Beans*
Ⓢ *Spiced Refried Beans* Ⓢ *Spicy Refried Beans* Ⓢ
Traditional Refried Beans Ⓢ *Vegan Refried Beans*

Sweetened or Flavored Legumes

Some pre-packaged legumes and pulses can have added sugars or high-sodium sauces and seasonings. For example, canned chickpeas in a sweetened sauce or black beans in a high-sodium taco mix might not be the best options.

⊘ Canned Legumes in Barbecue Sauce ⊘ Canned Legumes in Blueberry Sauce ⊘ Canned Legumes in Bourbon Sauce ⊘ Canned Legumes in Brown Sugar Glaze ⊘ Canned Legumes in Coconut Curry Sauce ⊘ Canned Legumes in Hoisin Sauce ⊘ Canned Legumes in Honey Lime Sauce ⊘ Canned Legumes in Honey Mustard Sauce ⊘ Canned Legumes in Mango Habanero Sauce ⊘ Canned Legumes in Mango Sauce ⊘ Canned Legumes in Maple BBQ Sauce ⊘ Canned Legumes in Orange Glaze ⊘ Canned Legumes in Peach Sauce ⊘ Canned Legumes in Pineapple Sauce ⊘ Canned Legumes in Pineapple Teriyaki Sauce ⊘ Canned Legumes in Raspberry Sauce ⊘ Canned Legumes in Strawberry Sauce ⊘ Canned Legumes in Sweet and Sour Sauce ⊘ Canned Legumes in Sweet and Spicy Sauce ⊘ Canned Legumes in Sweet and Tangy Sauce ⊘ Canned Legumes in Sweet Barbecue Sauce ⊘ Canned Legumes in Sweet Basil Sauce ⊘ Canned Legumes in Sweet Buffalo Sauce ⊘ Canned Legumes in Sweet Cajun Sauce ⊘ Canned Legumes in Sweet Chili Sauce ⊘ Canned Legumes in Sweet Chipotle Sauce ⊘ Canned Legumes in Sweet Cilantro Lime Sauce ⊘ Canned Legumes in Sweet Curry Sauce ⊘ Canned Legumes in Sweet Garlic Sauce ⊘ Canned Legumes in Sweet Ginger Sauce ⊘ Canned Legumes in Sweet Herb Sauce ⊘ Canned Legumes in Sweet Lemon Sauce ⊘ Canned Legumes in Sweet Mustard Sauce ⊘ Canned Legumes in Sweet Onion Sauce ⊘ Canned Legumes in Sweet Paprika Sauce ⊘ Canned Legumes in Sweet Pesto Sauce ⊘ Canned Legumes in Sweet Ranch Sauce ⊘ Canned Legumes in Sweet Sesame Sauce ⊘ Canned Legumes in Sweet Soy Sauce ⊘ Canned Legumes in Sweet

Sriracha Sauce ⊘ Canned Legumes in Sweet Sun-Dried
Tomato Sauce ⊘ Canned Legumes in Sweet
Worcestershire Sauce ⊘ Canned Legumes in Tomato
Sauce with Added Sugar ⊘ Canned Sweetened Baked
Beans ⊘ Flavored Canned Black Beans in Sauce ⊘
Honey-Glazed Canned Lentils ⊘ Maple Syrup Canned
Navy Beans ⊘ Sweet Chili Sauce Canned Kidney Beans
⊘ Sweetened Canned Chickpeas ⊘ Teriyaki-Flavored
Canned Edamame

. **Processed Pulses**: Products made from pulses, such as certain types
of crackers or snacks, usually contain other high-carb ingredients and
are lower in fiber.

⊘ Black Bean-based Breakfast Burritos with Added Flour
Tortillas ⊘ Black Bean-based Cookies with Added
Refined Wheat Flour ⊘ Black Bean-based Donuts with
Added Wheat Flour ⊘ Black Bean-based Pretzels with
Added Wheat Flour ⊘ Black Bean-based Rice Cakes with
Added Grain Fillers ⊘ Black Bean-based Veggie Sausages
with Added Fillers ⊘ Black Bean-based Waffles with
Added Starches ⊘ Chickpea-based Bread with Added
Wheat Flour ⊘ Chickpea-based Breakfast Cereals with
Added Artificial Sweeteners ⊘ Chickpea-based Breakfast
Cereals with Added Sugars ⊘ Chickpea-based Cereal
Bars with Added Artificial Colors ⊘ Chickpea-based
Cereal Bars with Added Sugars ⊘ Chickpea-based Chips
with Added Antioxidants ⊘ Chickpea-based Cookies with
Added Trans Fats ⊘ Chickpea-based Crackers with
Added Hydrogenated Oils ⊘ Chickpea-based Crackers
with Added Vegetable Oils ⊘ Chickpea-based Crackers
with Added Wheat Flour ⊘ Chickpea-based Donuts with
Added Artificial Coloring ⊘ Chickpea-based Pancake

Mix with Added Artificial Sweeteners ⊘ Chickpea-based Pancake Mix with Added Sugar Substitutes ⊘ Chickpea-based Pasta with Added Gluten ⊘ Chickpea-based Pita Chips with Added Artificial Sweeteners ⊘ Chickpea-based Pita Chips with Added White Flour ⊘ Chickpea-based Pizza Crust with Added Wheat Grains ⊘ Chickpea-based Pretzels with Added Preservatives ⊘ Chickpea-based Snack Bars with Added High-Fructose Corn Syrup ⊘ Chickpea-based Tortilla Chips with Added Cornmeal ⊘ Chickpea-based Tortilla Chips with Added MSG ⊘ Lentil-based Bread with Added Dough Conditioners ⊘ Lentil-based Chips with Added Artificial Flavorings ⊘ Lentil-based Chips with Added Maltodextrin ⊘ Lentil-based Chips with Added Potato Starch ⊘ Lentil-based Crackers with Added Emulsifiers ⊘ Lentil-based Granola Bars with Added Artificial Preservatives ⊘ Lentil-based Granola Bars with Added Sweeteners ⊘ Lentil-based Muffins with Added Artificial Flavors ⊘ Lentil-based Muffins with Added Refined Flours ⊘ Lentil-based Pancake Mix with Added All-Purpose Flour ⊘ Lentil-based Pasta with Added Enriched Wheat Flour ⊘ Lentil-based Pizza Crust with Added Yeast Enhancers ⊘ Lentil-based Puffs with Added Artificial Colorings ⊘ Lentil-based Rice Cakes with Added Artificial Additives ⊘ Lentil-based Snack Mix with Added High-Fructose Corn Syrup ⊘ Lentil-based Snack Mix with Added Wheat Cereals ⊘ Lentil-based Veggie Burgers with Added Bread Crumbs ⊘ Lentil-based Waffles with Added Cornstarch ⊘ Lentil-based Waffles with Added Fillers ⊘ Pea-based Puffs with Added Rice Cereal ⊘ Split Pea-based Crackers with Added Wheat Flour ⊘ Split Pea-based Pasta with Added Semolina Flour

* * *

In the subsequent section of this chapter, comprehensive tables are provided to outline foods that are non-compliant with Reverse Type 2 Diabetes Diet. These tables offer detailed information including serving size, Glycemic Index (GI), Glycemic Load (GL), and Net Carbohydrates for each food item. These metrics are particularly relevant when a food item's non-compliance is attributed to a high glycemic load and/or high carbohydrate content.

However, it is important to note that not all non-compliant foods can be categorized solely based on their GI, GL, or net carbohydrate content. Some food items are deemed non-compliant due to factors such as extensive processing, excessive sodium content, or an abundance of unhealthy fats. For these specific food items, detailed GI, GL, or net carb data may not be provided in the tables. Instead, they are simply listed with a note indicating their non-compliant status. This differentiation is aimed at ensuring clarity in understanding why certain food items are not recommended under the principles of the Reverse Type 2 Diabetes Diet.

LEGUMES & PULSES

LEGUMES	SERVING SIZE	GI	GL	NET CARB
Adzuki Beans, Canned, Regular	1 serving, 50g	Non-compliant foods		
Black Beans, Canned, Regular	1 serving, 50g	Non-compliant foods		
Black-eyed Peas, Canned, Regular	1 serving, 50g	Non-compliant foods		
Butter Beans, Canned, Regular	1 serving, 50g	Non-compliant foods		
Cannellini Beans, Canned, Regular	1 serving, 50g	Non-compliant foods		
Cranberry Beans, Canned, Regular	1 serving, 50g	Non-compliant foods		
Fava Beans, Canned, Regular	1 serving, 50g	Non-compliant foods		
Garbanzo Beans, Canned, Regular	1 serving, 50g	Non-compliant foods		
Great Northern Beans, Canned, Regular	1 serving, 50g	Non-compliant foods		
Green Snap Beans, Canned, Regular	1 serving, 50g	Non-compliant foods		
Green String Beans, Canned, Regular	1 serving, 50g	Non-compliant foods		
Highly processed Bean-based "Bacon"	1 serving, 50g	Non-compliant foods		
Highly processed Bean-based "Chicken"	1 serving, 50g	Non-compliant foods		
Highly processed Bean-based "Corned Beef"	1 serving, 50g	Non-compliant foods		
Highly processed Bean-based "Ham"	1 serving, 50g	Non-compliant foods		

LEGUMES	SERVING SIZE	GI	GL	NET CARB
Highly processed Bean-based "Pastrami"	1 serving, 50g	Non-compliant foods		
Highly processed Bean-based "Pepperoni"	1 serving, 50g	Non-compliant foods		
Highly processed Bean-based "Roast Beef"	1 serving, 50g	Non-compliant foods		
Highly processed Bean-based "Salami"	1 serving, 50g	Non-compliant foods		
Highly processed Bean-based "Turkey"	1 serving, 50g	Non-compliant foods		
Highly processed Veggie Burgers	1 serving, 50g	Non-compliant foods		
Kidney Beans, Canned, Regular	1 serving, 50g	Non-compliant foods		
Lentils, Canned, Regular	1 serving, 50g	Non-compliant foods		
Lima Beans, Canned, Regular	1 serving, 50g	Non-compliant foods		
Mung Beans, Canned, Regular	1 serving, 50g	Non-compliant foods		
Navy Beans, Canned, Regular	1 serving, 50g	Non-compliant foods		
Pinto Beans, Canned, Regular	1 serving, 50g	Non-compliant foods		
Red Beans, Canned, Regular	1 serving, 50g	Non-compliant foods		
Soybeans, Canned, Regular	1 serving, 50g	Non-compliant foods		
Sweetened Azuki Beans	1 serving, 50g	High	High	Varies
Sweetened Black-Eyed Peas	1 serving, 50g	High	High	Varies
Sweetened Cannellini Beans	1 serving, 50g	High	High	Varies
Sweetened Chickpeas	1 serving, 50g	High	High	Varies
Sweetened Great Northern Beans	1 serving, 50g	High	High	Varies

LEGUMES	SERVING SIZE	GI	GL	NET CARB
Sweetened Kidney Beans	1 serving, 50g	High	High	Varies
Sweetened Lentils	1 serving, 50g	High	High	Varies
Sweetened Lima Beans	1 serving, 50g	High	High	Varies
Sweetened Mung Beans	1 serving, 50g	High	High	Varies
Sweetened Navy Beans	1 serving, 50g	High	High	Varies
Sweetened Pinto Beans	1 serving, 50g	High	High	Varies
Sweetened Red Beans	1 serving, 50g	High	High	Varies
Sweetened Soybeans	1 serving, 50g	High	High	Varies

BEVERAGES AND DRINKS

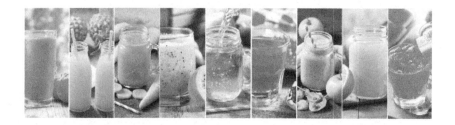

A variety of beverages and drinks, while tempting, are often incompatible with the principles of a Type 2 Diabetes (T2D) reversal diet, which combines Glycemic Load (GL) guidelines, the Mediterranean Diet (MedDiet), 2020-2025 Dietary Guidelines for Americans, and 17 principles of a healthy, balanced diet.

Sugary Drinks and Sodas: These are often high in added sugars and provide little to no nutritional value. They can cause rapid blood sugar spikes and contribute significantly to excess caloric intake, both of which can exacerbate T2D. They clearly do not align with the low GL, balanced nutrient intake, and limited sugar intake principles of the Reverse Type 2 Diabetes Diet.

Fruit Juices: Even when freshly squeezed or labeled as 100% juice, fruit juices can pose a problem. They contain concentrated natural sugars and lack the fiber found in whole fruit. This combination can lead to rapid blood glucose increases, and they don't promote satiety as effectively as whole fruits. As such, fruit juices typically contravene the principles of a balanced glycemic response and sufficient fiber intake, fundamental to Reverse Type 2 Diabetes Diet.

Alcoholic Beverages: Consuming alcohol excessively can contribute to weight gain and cause instability in blood sugar levels. Alcoholic drinks can also interfere with certain diabetes medications, making it difficult to manage T2D effectively. While the MedDiet includes moderate wine consumption, the key is moderation and not all types of alcoholic beverages are advisable.

Sweetened Teas and Coffees: While tea and coffee themselves are not an issue, the addition of sugars, syrups, and creamers can make them less suitable. The extra calories and sugars in these additives can spike blood glucose levels and contribute to weight gain. They don't conform with the low GL and low added sugars guidelines central to Reverse Type 2 Diabetes Diet.

Energy and Sports Drinks: Often packed with sugars and caffeine, these beverages can cause a quick surge and subsequent drop in blood sugar levels, which can be problematic for T2D management. They're typically high in calories and offer little nutritional benefit, conflicting with the principles of balanced nutrient intake and controlled caloric intake.

Instead of these drinks, opt for water, unsweetened teas, and occasionally moderate amounts of coffee (without sweeteners or unhealthy creamers). When drinking alcohol, moderation is key, and the best choices are generally wine or light beer. Remember, the goal is to avoid rapid blood glucose spikes and unnecessary caloric intake, maintaining a balance of nutrients in line with Reverse Type 2 Diabetes Diet principles.

* * *

In the subsequent section of this chapter, comprehensive tables are provided to outline foods that are non-compliant with Reverse Type 2 Diabetes Diet. These tables offer detailed information including serving size, Glycemic Index (GI), Glycemic Load (GL), and Net Carbohydrates for each food item. These metrics are particularly relevant when a food item's non-compliance is attributed to a high glycemic load and/or high carbohydrate content.

However, it is important to note that not all non-compliant foods can be categorized solely based on their GI, GL, or net carbohydrate content. Some food items are deemed non-compliant due to factors such as extensive processing, excessive sodium content, or an abundance of unhealthy fats. For these specific food items, detailed GI, GL, or net carb data may not be provided in the tables. Instead, they are simply listed with a note indicating their non-compliant status. This differentiation is aimed at ensuring clarity in understanding why certain food items are not recommended under the principles of the Reverse Type 2 Diabetes Diet.

BEVERAGES & DRINKS

BEVERAGES & DRINKS	SERVING SIZE	GI	GL	NET CARB
Banana Milkshake	1 cup (240ml)	66	39.6	60g
Birch Beer	1 cup (240ml)	68	23.1	34g
Bubble (Boba) Tea	1 cup (240ml)	70	42	60g
Caramel Frappuccino	1 cup (240ml)	45	30.2	67g
Carbonated Lemonade	1 cup (240ml)	72	21.6	30g
Chocolate Banana Smoothie	1 cup (240ml)	45	30.6	68g
Cola	1 cup (240ml)	63	16.4	26g
Commercial Dairy Drinks Regular	-	Non-compliant foods		
Commercial Flavored Coffee Drinks	-	Non-compliant foods		
Commercial Frappuccino's Made	-	Non-compliant foods		
Commercial Fruit Drink Made	-	Non-compliant foods		
Commercial Fruit Juice Made	-	Non-compliant foods		
Commercial Vegetable Drink Made	-	Non-compliant foods		
Commercial Vegetables Juice Made	-	Non-compliant foods		
Cookies and Cream Milkshake	1 cup (240ml)	60	48	80g
Cream Soda	1 cup (240ml)	71	21.3	30g
Dr. Pepper	1 cup (240ml)	72	19.4	27g
Energy Drink (regular)	1 cup (240ml)	72	20.2	28g
Energy Drinks	-	Non-compliant foods		

BEVERAGES & DRINKS	SERVING SIZE	GI	GL	NET CARB
Energy Shot	1 cup (240ml)	70	21	30g
Fanta	1 cup (240ml)	72	20.2	28g
Flavored Waters with Added Sugars	-	Non-compliant foods		
Frappuccino	1 cup (240ml)	50	25	50g
Fruit Punch	1 cup (240ml)	67	18.8	28g
Ginger Ale	1 cup (240ml)	63	16.4	26g
Ginger Beer	1 cup (240ml)	60	24	40g
Grape Soda	1 cup (240ml)	63	25.2	40g
Horchata	1 cup (240ml)	70	30.1	43g
Hot Chocolate	1 cup (240ml)	60	18	30g
Hot Chocolate with Whipped Cream	1 cup (240ml)	63	22.1	35g
Hot Cider	1 cup (240ml)	65	16.9	26g
Iced Caramel Latte	1 cup (240ml)	60	21.6	36g
Iced Mocha	1 cup (240ml)	63	22.1	35g
Iced Vanilla Latte	1 cup (240ml)	60	19.8	33g
Lemon-Lime Soda	1 cup (240ml)	63	16.4	26g
Long Island Iced Tea	1 cup (240ml)	70	30.8	44g
Malted Milk	1 cup (240ml)	50	22.5	45g
Milkshakes with Added Sugars	-	Non-compliant foods		
Mocha	1 cup (240ml)	55	22	40g
Mocha Frappuccino	1 cup (240ml)	65	42.3	65g
Mountain Dew	1 cup (240ml)	63	19.5	31g
Oat Milk, sweetened	1 cup (240ml)	70	16.8	24g
Orange Soda	1 cup (240ml)	63	19.5	31g
Peach Milkshake	1 cup (240ml)	40	28	70g
Pepsi	1 cup (240ml)	63	16.4	26g

BEVERAGES & DRINKS	SERVING SIZE	GI	GL	NET CARB
Pina Colada	1 cup (240ml)	70	22.4	32g
Pre-packaged Iced Tea	-	Non-compliant foods		
Pumpkin Spice Latte	1 cup (240ml)	70	36.4	52g
Rice Milk	1 cup (240ml)	86	18.9	22g
Rice Milk, sweetened	1 cup (240ml)	91	27.3	30g
Root Beer	1 cup (240ml)	63	18.9	30g
Smoothies with Added Sugars	-	Non-compliant foods		
Soda Regular	-	Non-compliant foods		
Spiced Pumpkin Latte	1 cup (240ml)	70	35	50g
Sports Drink (regular)	1 cup (240ml)	78	10.9	14g
Sports Drinks with added sugars.	-	Non-compliant foods		
Sprite	1 cup (240ml)	63	16.4	26g
Strawberry Milkshake	1 cup (240ml)	30	18	60g
Sweetened Condensed Milk	1 cup (240ml)	61	101.3	166g
Sweetened Iced Tea	-	Non-compliant foods		
Sweetened Plant-Based Milk Alternatives	-	Non-compliant foods		
Vanilla Milkshake	1 cup (240ml)	35	21	60g
White Chocolate Mocha	1 cup (240ml)	43	25.8	60g
White Hot Chocolate	1 cup (240ml)	50	20	40g
Sweetened Iced Tea	-	Non-compliant foods		
Sweetened Plant-Based Milk Alternatives	-	Non-compliant foods		
Vanilla Milkshake	1 cup (240ml)	35	21	60g

DAIRY AND PLANT-BASED ALTERNATIVES

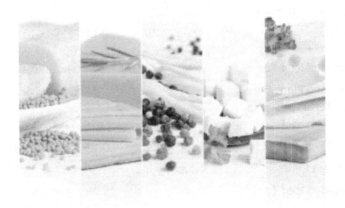

Adhering to a Type 2 Diabetes (T2D) reversal diet, which combines the Glycemic Load (GL) framework, the Mediterranean Diet (MedDiet), 2020-2025 Dietary Guidelines for Americans (DGA), and 17 principles of a healthy, balanced diet, requires careful selection of dairy and plant-based alternatives.

Sweetened Dairy Products: Foods like flavored yogurts, sweetened milk, and processed cheese often contain added sugars that can lead to rapid increases in blood glucose levels, which contravene the GL guidelines of the Reverse Type 2 Diabetes Diet. Moreover, these products often contain unhealthy fats, preservatives, and other additives that defy the MedDiet's emphasis on natural, minimally processed foods.

Full-Fat Dairy Products: While dairy can be a valuable source of protein and calcium, full-fat versions such as whole milk, cream, and full-fat cheeses can lead to excessive intake of saturated fats, conflicting with the DGA's recommendations for heart health. High-fat dairy products can also contribute to weight gain, making T2D management more challenging.

Sweetened Plant-Based Milk Alternatives: While plant-based milk alternatives can be good options, those that are sweetened or flavored often contain added sugars, causing spikes in blood sugar levels. They may also lack the nutritional value of their unsweetened counterparts, as they may not be fortified with essential vitamins and minerals. These products do not align with the GL framework and balanced nutrition principles of the Reverse Type 2 Diabetes Diet:

◊ Flavored almond-based yogurt drinks/smoothies ◊ Flavored coconut-based butter/margarine ◊ Flavored coconut-based coffee creamer ◊ Flavored coconut-based cream cheese ◊ Flavored coconut-based ice cream ◊ Flavored coconut-based sour cream ◊ Flavored coconut-based whipped cream ◊ Flavored coconut-based yogurt ◊ Flavored flax milk ◊ Flavored hemp milk ◊ Flavored oat milk ◊ Flavored oat-based yogurt ◊ Flavored oat-based yogurt drinks/smoothies ◊ Flavored soy-based yogurt drinks/smoothies ◊ Sweetened almond milk ◊ Sweetened almond-based butter/margarine ◊ Sweetened almond-based cheese spreads/dips ◊ Sweetened almond-based coffee creamer ◊ Sweetened

almond-based cream cheese ⊘ *Sweetened almond-based ice cream* ⊘ *Sweetened almond-based sour cream* ⊘ *Sweetened almond-based whipped cream* ⊘ *Sweetened almond-based yogurt* ⊘ *Sweetened cashew milk* ⊘ *Sweetened cashew-based yogurt* ⊘ *Sweetened coconut milk* ⊘ *Sweetened coconut-based yogurt drinks/smoothies* ⊘ *Sweetened hazelnut milk* ⊘ *Sweetened macadamia nut milk* ⊘ *Sweetened oat-based butter/margarine* ⊘ *Sweetened oat-based coffee creamer* ⊘ *Sweetened oat-based cream cheese* ⊘ *Sweetened oat-based sour cream* ⊘ *Sweetened oat-based whipped cream* ⊘ *Sweetened pea milk* ⊘ *Sweetened rice milk* ⊘ *Sweetened rice-based ice cream* ⊘ *Sweetened soy milk* ⊘ *Sweetened soy-based butter/margarine* ⊘ *Sweetened soy-based coffee creamer* ⊘ *Sweetened soy-based cream cheese* ⊘ *Sweetened soy-based ice cream* ⊘ *Sweetened soy-based sour cream* ⊘ *Sweetened soy-based whipped cream* ⊘ *Sweetened soy-based yogurt* ⊘ *Sweetened walnut milk*

Highly Processed Plant-Based Alternatives: Many plant-based products undergo extensive processing and often contain added sugars, unhealthy fats, and elevated sodium levels. For instance, some vegan cheeses and meat substitutes fall into this category. These items do not conform to the MedDiet and 2020-2025 Dietary Guidelines for Americans for low sodium intake, minimally processed foods, and balanced nutrient intake:

⊘ *Plant-based butter* ⊘ *Plant-based cheese blocks/wheels* ⊘ *Plant-based cheese dips/spreads* ⊘ *Plant-based cheese sauces* ⊘ *Plant-based cheese slices* ⊘ *Plant-based cheese spreads/dips* ⊘ *Plant-based cheese-filled breadsticks* ⊘ *Plant-based cheese-filled pasta (e.g., vegan stuffed shells, vegan ravioli)* ⊘ *Plant-based cheese-filled pastries (e.g., vegan cheese danishes, vegan cheese croissants)* Ⓢ *Plant-based cheese-filled pretzels* Ⓢ *Plant-based cheese-filled quesadillas* Ⓢ *Plant-based cheese-filled sandwiches/burgers* Ⓢ *Plant-based cheese-filled snacks (e.g., vegan cheese puffs, vegan cheese balls)* Ⓢ *Plant-based cheese-filled tarts* Ⓢ *Plant-based cheese-filled wraps/burritos* Ⓢ *Plant-based cheese-flavored biscuits* Ⓢ *Plant-based cheese-flavored bread* Ⓢ *Plant-based cheese-flavored breaded products (e.g., vegan cheese sticks, vegan cheese bites)* Ⓢ *Plant-based cheese-flavored crackers* Ⓢ *Plant-based cheese-flavored crackers/chips* Ⓢ *Plant-based cheese-flavored crackers/crisps* Ⓢ *Plant-based cheese-flavored dips for chips/crackers* Ⓢ *Plant-based cheese-flavored dips for vegetables/crackers* Ⓢ *Plant-based cheese-flavored dressings for salads* Ⓢ *Plant-based cheese-flavored dressings for sandwiches/wraps* Ⓢ *Plant-based cheese-flavored frozen appetizers (e.g., vegan cheese sticks, vegan cheese bites)* Ⓢ *Plant-based cheese-flavored instant meals* Ⓢ *Plant-based cheese-flavored popcorn* Ⓢ *Plant-based cheese-flavored popcorn seasoning* Ⓢ *Plant-based cheese-flavored protein bars* Ⓢ *Plant-based cheese-flavored puffs/corn snacks* Ⓢ *Plant-based cheese-flavored rice cakes* Ⓢ *Plant-based cheese-flavored rice/pasta dishes* Ⓢ *Plant-based cheese-flavored salad dressings* Ⓢ *Plant-based cheese-flavored sauces for nachos* Ⓢ *Plant-based cheese-flavored sauces for pasta* Ⓢ *Plant-based cheese-flavored seasoning mixes* Ⓢ *Plant-based cheese-flavored seasonings for popcorn/fries* Ⓢ *Plant-based cheese-flavored snack bars* Ⓢ *Plant-based cheese-flavored vegetable chips* Ⓢ *Plant-based cheese-flavored vegetable spreads* Ⓢ *Plant-based cheese-stuffed crusts (e.g., vegan stuffed crust pizza)* Ⓢ *Plant-based chocolate milk* Ⓢ *Plant-based coffee creamers* Ⓢ *Plant-based condensed milk* Ⓢ *Plant-based cream cheese* Ⓢ *Plant-based cream-filled pastries (e.g., sweetened vegan cream puffs)* Ⓢ

Plant-based creamer for cooking/baking ⊘ *Plant-based creamer for desserts* ⊘ *Plant-based creamer for soups/sauces* ⊘ *Plant-based creamers for tea/hot beverages* ⊘ *Plant-based custards/puddings* ⊘ *Plant-based frozen yogurt* ⊘ *Plant-based half-and-half* ⊘ *Plant-based ice cream* ⊘ *Plant-based margarine* ⊘ *Plant-based milkshakes* ⊘ *Plant-based smoothies* ⊘ *Plant-based sour cream* ⊘ *Plant-based whipped cream* ⊘ *Plant-based whipped toppings* ⊘ *Plant-based whipped toppings for desserts* ⊘ *Plant-based yogurt drinks* ⊘ *Vegan cheddar shreds (with preservatives or additives)* ⊘ *Vegan cheese bites (with preservatives or additives)* ⊘ *Vegan cheese sticks (with preservatives or additives)* ⊘ *Vegan mozzarella shreds (with preservatives or additives)*

Instead, opt for unsweetened, low-fat, or non-fat dairy products and unsweetened, fortified plant-based alternatives. These options align better with the principles of a healthy, balanced diet, as they offer essential nutrients without the adverse effects of high sugar, unhealthy fats, and high sodium content.

In the subsequent section of this chapter, comprehensive tables are provided to outline foods that are non-compliant with Reverse Type 2 Diabetes Diet. These tables offer detailed information including serving size, Glycemic Index (GI), Glycemic Load (GL), and Net Carbohydrates for each food item. These metrics are particularly relevant when a food item's non-compliance is attributed to a high glycemic load and/or high carbohydrate content.

However, it is important to note that not all non-compliant foods can be categorized solely based on their GI, GL, or net carbohydrate content. Some food items are deemed non-compliant due to factors such as extensive processing, excessive sodium content, or an abundance of unhealthy fats. For these specific food items, detailed GI, GL, or net carb data may not be provided in the tables. Instead, they are simply listed with a note indicating their non-compliant status. This differentiation is aimed at ensuring clarity in understanding why certain food items are not recommended under the principles of the Reverse Type 2 Diabetes Diet.

DAIRY & PLANT-BASED ALTERNATIVES

DAIRY & PLANT-BASED ALTERNATIVES	
Blue Cheese	Non-compliant foods
American cheese slices	Non-compliant foods
Annie's Macaroni & Cheese	Non-compliant foods
Banoffee Pie	Non-compliant foods
Betty Crocker Macaroni & Cheese	Non-compliant foods
Brigadeiro	Non-compliant foods
Cheddar cheese slices	Non-compliant foods
Cheez Whiz	Non-compliant foods
Coconut Ice	Non-compliant foods
Coconut Macadamia Balls	Non-compliant foods
Coconut Macaroons	Non-compliant foods
Colby Jack cheese slices	Non-compliant foods
Crystal Farms Shredded Cheese	Non-compliant foods
Crystal Farms String Cheese	Non-compliant foods
Dessert-Style Plant-Based Puddings	Non-compliant foods
Easy Cheese	Non-compliant foods
Feta Cheese	Non-compliant foods
Flan/Caramel Custard	Non-compliant foods
Flavored Milk	Non-compliant foods
Flavored Plant-Based Yogurts	Non-compliant foods
Flavored Plant-Based Yogurts	Non-compliant foods
Flavored Soy Milk	Non-compliant foods
Flavored Yogurt	Non-compliant foods
Frigo Cheese Heads String Cheese	Non-compliant foods
Fritos Jalapeno Cheddar Cheese Dip	Non-compliant foods

DAIRY & PLANT-BASED ALTERNATIVES

Fruit Yogurt Parfaits	Non-compliant foods
Fudge	Non-compliant foods
Fudge Brownies	Non-compliant foods
Galbani String Cheese	Non-compliant foods
Gorgonzola Cheese	Non-compliant foods
Halloumi Cheese	Non-compliant foods
Heluva Good French Onion Dip (with cheese flavor)	Non-compliant foods
Herr's Cheese Curls Cheese Dip	Non-compliant foods
Horizon Organic Mozzarella String Cheese	Non-compliant foods
Ice cream	Non-compliant foods
Icebox Cake	Non-compliant foods
Key Lime Pie	Non-compliant foods
Kraft Easy Cheese Cheddar 'n Bacon Cheese Dip	Non-compliant foods
Kraft Macaroni & Cheese	Non-compliant foods
Kraft Mozzarella String Cheese	Non-compliant foods
Kraft Shredded Cheese	Non-compliant foods
Lemon Bars	Non-compliant foods
Magic Bars	Non-compliant foods
Maruchan Instant Macaroni and Cheese	Non-compliant foods
Milkshakes	Non-compliant foods
Nacho Cheese Sauce	Non-compliant foods
Old El Paso Queso Dip	Non-compliant foods
Organic Valley Shredded Cheese	Non-compliant foods
Parmesan Cheese	Non-compliant foods
Pecorino Romano Cheese	Non-compliant foods
Plant-Based Creamers	Non-compliant foods
Plant-Based Dessert Alternatives	Non-compliant foods
Polly-O String Cheese	Non-compliant foods

DAIRY & PLANT-BASED ALTERNATIVES	
Processed Cheese	Non-compliant foods
Provolone cheese slices	Non-compliant foods
Ricos Cheese Sauce	Non-compliant foods
Ricos Gourmet Nacho Cheese Sauce	Non-compliant foods
Roquefort Cheese	Non-compliant foods
Sargento Shredded Cheese	Non-compliant foods
Sargento String Cheese	Non-compliant foods
Sweet Cream Cheese Spreads	Non-compliant foods
Sweetened Almond Milk	Non-compliant foods
Sweetened Cashew Milk	Non-compliant foods
Sweetened Coconut Milk	Non-compliant foods
Sweetened Condensed Milk	Non-compliant foods
Sweetened Oat Milk	Non-compliant foods
Sweetened Plant-Based Creamers	Non-compliant foods
Sweetened Rice Milk	Non-compliant foods
Sweetened Whipped Cream	Non-compliant foods
Tillamook Shredded Cheese	Non-compliant foods
Tostitos Cheese Dip	Non-compliant foods
Tostitos Queso Blanco Dip	Non-compliant foods
Trader Joe's Shredded Cheese	Non-compliant foods
Tres Leches Cake	Non-compliant foods
Vegan Cheese Alternatives	Non-compliant foods
Velveeta	Non-compliant foods
Velveeta Shells & Cheese	Non-compliant foods
Vietnamese Coffee	Non-compliant foods

DIPS AND DRESSINGS

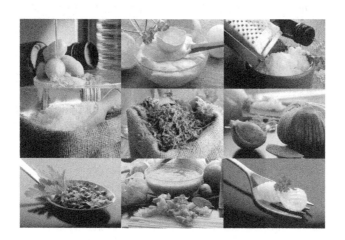

Many dips and dressings, while seemingly innocuous, may not align with a Type 2 Diabetes (T2D) reversal diet. This diet merges the Glycemic Load (GL) framework, the Mediterranean Diet (MedDiet), 2020-2025 Dietary Guidelines for Americans, and 17 principles of a healthy, balanced diet.

CREAMY AND FULL-FAT DRESSINGS

Dressings such as ranch, blue cheese, and thousand island are commonly known for their high levels of saturated fats and calories. Consuming these dressings in excess can potentially lead to weight gain and elevated blood glucose levels. Dressings that do not align with the low GL, reduced calorie, and low saturated fat principles of the Reverse Type 2 Diabetes Diet include:

Ⓢ *Avocado ranch dressing* Ⓢ *Blue cheese dressing* Ⓢ *Buttermilk dressing* Ⓢ *Caesar dressing* Ⓢ *Chipotle ranch dressing* Ⓢ *Creamy avocado cilantro dressing* Ⓢ *Creamy avocado lime dressing* Ⓢ *Creamy avocado ranch dressing* Ⓢ *Creamy bacon dressing* Ⓢ *Creamy bacon honey mustard dressing* Ⓢ *Creamy bacon ranch dressing* Ⓢ *Creamy balsamic dressing* Ⓢ *Creamy blue cheese dressing with added chunks of blue cheese* Ⓢ *Creamy blue cheese dressing with added ingredients (e.g., bacon, nuts)* Ⓢ *Creamy buffalo blue cheese dressing* Ⓢ *Creamy buffalo dressing* Ⓢ *Creamy buttermilk herb dressing* Ⓢ *Creamy buttermilk ranch dressing* Ⓢ *Creamy Caesar dressing* Ⓢ *Creamy Caesar dressing with added parmesan cheese* Ⓢ *Creamy chipotle lime dressing* Ⓢ *Creamy cilantro jalapeno dressing* Ⓢ *Creamy cilantro lime dressing* Ⓢ *Creamy coconut dressing* Ⓢ *Creamy cucumber dill dressing* Ⓢ *Creamy curry dressing* Ⓢ *Creamy dill dressing* Ⓢ *Creamy dill pickle dressing* Ⓢ *Creamy feta dill dressing* Ⓢ *Creamy garlic dressing* Ⓢ *Creamy garlic parmesan dressing* Ⓢ *Creamy ginger dressing* Ⓢ *Creamy Greek dressing* Ⓢ *Creamy honey mustard bacon dressing* Ⓢ *Creamy honey mustard dressing* Ⓢ *Creamy honey sesame dressing* Ⓢ *Creamy horseradish blue cheese dressing* Ⓢ *Creamy horseradish dressing* Ⓢ *Creamy Italian dressing* Ⓢ *Creamy lemon garlic tahini dressing* Ⓢ *Creamy lemon herb dressing* Ⓢ *Creamy miso dressing*

◎ *Creamy parmesan dressing* ◎ *Creamy peanut dressing* ◎ *Creamy pesto dressing* ◎ *Creamy poppy seed dressing* ◎ *Creamy roasted garlic dressing* ◎ *Creamy roasted red pepper dressing* ◎ *Creamy roasted red pepper feta dressing* ◎ *Creamy Sriracha dressing* ◎ *Creamy Sriracha lime dressing* ◎ *Creamy sun-dried tomato dressing* ◎ *Creamy tahini dressing* ◎ *Creamy walnut cranberry dressing* ◎ *Creamy walnut dressing* ◎ *French dressing (creamy variant)* ◎ *Honey mustard dressing (creamy variant)* ◎ *Ranch dressing* ◎ *Russian dressing* ◎ *Thousand Island dressing*

Sugary Dressings: Some dressings, including certain types of vinaigrettes and sweet dressings like honey mustard, can be high in added sugars. Consuming these dressings can result in rapid blood sugar spikes, which is a factor of non-compliance with the GL framework of the Reverse Type 2 Diabetes Diet.

◎ *Apricot vinaigrette* ◎ *Asian sesame dressing* ◎ *Balsamic glaze* ◎ *Banana dressing* ◎ *Blackberry vinaigrette* ◎ *Blueberry dressing* ◎ *Brown sugar bacon dressing* ◎ *Brown sugar bourbon dressing* ◎ *Brown sugar dressing* ◎ *Candied pecan dressing* ◎ *Caramelized onion dressing* ◎ *Cherry vinaigrette* ◎ *Cinnamon honey dressing* ◎ *Coconut lime dressing* ◎ *Cranberry vinaigrette* ◎ *Creamy blue cheese dressing with sweet additions* ◎ *Creamy candied bacon dressing* ◎ *Creamy caramel apple dressing* ◎ *Creamy caramelized onion dressing* ◎ *Creamy coconut lime dressing* ◎ *Creamy fruit dressing* ◎ *Creamy honey balsamic dressing* ◎ *Creamy honey chipotle dressing* ◎ *Creamy honey lime dressing* ◎ *Creamy honey mustard dressing* ◎ *Creamy honey sesame dressing* ◎ *Creamy honey sriracha dressing*

⊘ Creamy pecan praline dressing ⊘ Creamy raspberry walnut dressing ⊘ Fig balsamic dressing ⊘ French dressing ⊘ Grape dressing ⊘ Grapefruit vinaigrette ⊘ Hibiscus dressing ⊘ Honey almond dressing ⊘ Honey mustard dressing ⊘ Key lime dressing ⊘ Lemon poppy seed dressing ⊘ Lemonade dressing ⊘ Mango vinaigrette ⊘ Maple bacon vinaigrette ⊘ Maple pecan vinaigrette ⊘ Maple vinaigrette ⊘ Orange ginger dressing ⊘ Peach vinaigrette ⊘ Pineapple dressing ⊘ Pomegranate dressing ⊘ Poppy seed dressing ⊘ Raspberry chipotle dressing ⊘ Raspberry vinaigrette ⊘ Strawberry dressing ⊘ Sweet and creamy avocado lime dressing ⊘ Sweet and creamy bacon ranch dressing ⊘ Sweet and creamy pecan maple dressing ⊘ Sweet and creamy poppy seed dressing ⊘ Sweet and creamy sesame ginger dressing ⊘ Sweet and sour dressing ⊘ Sweet and tangy ranch dressing ⊘ Sweet chili sauce ⊘ Sweet onion dressing ⊘ Teriyaki glaze ⊘ Thousand Island dressing ⊘ Vanilla bean dressing ⊘ Watermelon vinaigrette

PROCESSED DIPS (COMMERCIALLY MADE)

Many commercially available dips, such as some varieties of salsa, queso, and spinach dip, can be heavily processed and high in sodium. They may also contain added sugars and unhealthy fats. The high sodium content and the processed nature of these dips make them incompatible with the MedDiet and DGA's emphasis on lower sodium and minimally processed foods. These products include:

⊘ Artichoke and parmesan dip ⊘ Artichoke and spinach dip ⊘ Bacon and cheddar dip ⊘ Bacon ranch dip ⊘ Barbecue bacon dip ⊘ BBQ ranch dip ⊘ Black bean dip ⊘ Buffalo cauliflower dip ⊘ Buffalo chicken dip ⊘ Buffalo ranch dip ⊘ Caramel apple dip ⊘ Caramelized onion dip ⊘ Cheeseburger dip ⊘ Cheesy spinach dip ⊘

Chili cheese dip Ⓢ Chipotle bacon dip Ⓢ Chocolate chip cookie dough dip Ⓢ Cilantro lime dip Ⓢ Crab dip Ⓢ Crab Rangoon dip Ⓢ Creamy dill dip Ⓢ Cucumber and dill dip Ⓢ Dill pickle dip Ⓢ Fiesta cheese dip Ⓢ French onion dip Ⓢ Greek tzatziki dip Ⓢ Honey mustard dip Ⓢ Honey sriracha dip Ⓢ Horseradish dip Ⓢ Hot bacon dip Ⓢ Jalapeno cheese dip Ⓢ Jalapeno popper dip Ⓢ Lemon herb dip Ⓢ Loaded baked potato dip Ⓢ Loaded nacho dip Ⓢ Mango salsa dip Ⓢ Olive tapenade dip Ⓢ Pepperoni pizza dip Ⓢ Pimento cheese dip Ⓢ Queso dip Ⓢ Ranch dip Ⓢ Roasted eggplant dip Ⓢ Roasted garlic dip Ⓢ Roasted red pepper dip Ⓢ S'mores dip Ⓢ Salsa con queso dip Ⓢ Seven-layer dip Ⓢ Smoked salmon dip Ⓢ Smoky chipotle dip Ⓢ Sour cream and onion dip Ⓢ Southwest fiesta dip Ⓢ Spicy avocado dip Ⓢ Spicy buffalo dip Ⓢ Spinach and artichoke dip Ⓢ Sriracha dip Ⓢ Sun-dried tomato dip Ⓢ Sweet and spicy mustard dip Ⓢ Sweet chili dip Ⓢ Tomato and basil dip Ⓢ White bean dip

Cheese-Based Dips: While delicious, these dips are often high in saturated fats and calories, which can contribute to weight gain and may affect blood glucose levels. They do not typically conform to the principles of balanced nutrient intake and reduced saturated fat content inherent to Reverse Type 2 Diabetes Diet.

Ⓢ Asiago and roasted garlic dip Ⓢ Asiago and sun-dried tomato dip Ⓢ Bacon and cheddar dip Ⓢ Beer cheese dip Ⓢ Blue cheese and bacon dip Ⓢ Blue cheese and walnut dip Ⓢ Blue cheese dip Ⓢ Boursin cheese dip Ⓢ Brie and cranberry dip Ⓢ Brie and honey dip Ⓢ Buffalo chicken dip Ⓢ Camembert and cranberry dip Ⓢ Camembert and fig dip Ⓢ Cheddar and beer dip Ⓢ Cheddar and green onion dip Ⓢ Cheesy bacon dip Ⓢ Cheesy buffalo dip Ⓢ Chili cheese dip Ⓢ Chipotle cheese dip Ⓢ Colby and horseradish dip Ⓢ Colby Jack dip Ⓢ Creamy feta dip Ⓢ

335

Edam and chive dip ◎ Feta and roasted red pepper dip ◎
Feta and spinach dip ◎ Fontina and mushroom dip ◎
Fontina and roasted pepper dip ◎ Fontina and spinach
dip ◎ Four cheese dip ◎ Garlic and herb cheese dip ◎
Goat cheese and apricot dip ◎ Gorgonzola and
caramelized onion dip ◎ Gorgonzola dip ◎ Gouda and
caramelized onion dip ◎ Gruyere and bacon dip ◎
Gruyere and caramelized onion dip ◎ Havarti and dill
dip ◎ Havarti and sun-dried tomato dip ◎ Havarti and
sun-dried tomato dip ◎ Horseradish cheddar dip ◎
Jalapeno popper dip ◎ Mexican queso dip ◎ Monterey
Jack and jalapeno dip ◎ Monterey Jack dip ◎
Mozzarella and basil dip ◎ Mozzarella and pesto dip ◎
Parmesan and artichoke dip ◎ Parmesan and black
pepper dip ◎ Pepper Jack and bacon dip ◎ Pepper Jack
and habanero dip ◎ Pepper Jack and jalapeno dip ◎
Pepper Jack dip ◎ Pimento cheese dip ◎ Provolone and
Italian herbs dip ◎ Provolone and roasted red pepper dip
◎ Queso dip ◎ Ranch dip ◎ Ricotta and herb dip ◎
Ricotta and roasted garlic dip ◎ Roquefort and walnut
dip ◎ Roquefort dip ◎ Smoked cheddar dip ◎ Smoked
Gouda and bacon dip ◎ Smoked Gouda and chipotle dip
◎ Smoked Gouda dip ◎ Spinach and cheese dip ◎
Stilton and walnut dip ◎ Swiss and caramelized onion
dip ◎ Swiss and mushroom dip ◎ Swiss cheese dip

Instead of these non-compliant options, opt for healthier dips and dressings. Consider homemade vinaigrettes made with olive oil, vinegar, and herbs, or dips made from Greek yogurt or mashed avocado. Hummus can also be a healthy option. These choices can offer the flavor and texture you seek without the negative impacts on your blood sugar and overall health. As always, moderation is key even with healthier choices.

GRAINS, CEREALS AND PASTA

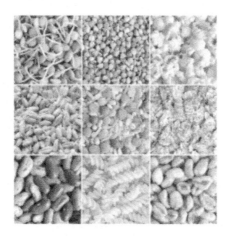

Grains, cereals, and pasta are staples in many diets around the world, providing essential nutrients, energy, and a comforting element to meals. However, there are certain considerations when it comes to these carbohydrate-rich foods in the context of reversing Type 2 Diabetes (T2D). Factors such as their high glycemic index (GI), high glycemic load (GL), removal of fiber through processing, and the presence of added sugars and sodium need to be taken into account. Here are some categories that do not comply with the diet's principles.

- **Refined Grains:** Refined grains, including white bread, white rice, and conventional pasta, undergo extensive processing that removes the fiber and nutrient-rich outer layers. This refining process results in easily digestible carbohydrates that quickly raise blood glucose levels after consumption. For individuals aiming to control or reverse T2D, these refined grains are not an option.

- **Sugary Cereals:** Many breakfast cereals available in supermarkets are loaded with added sugars, making them unsuitable for a Reverse Type 2 Diabetes Diet. These cereals often lack sufficient fiber and protein content to slow down digestion and prevent rapid blood sugar spikes. Therefore, it is important to carefully read product labels, select cereals with minimal added sugars, and explore healthier breakfast alternatives.

- **Flavored Instant Oatmeal:** While flavored instant oatmeal may appear convenient and delicious, they often contain excessive amounts of added sugars and artificial flavorings. These additives undermine the nutritional value of the oats. Opting for plain oats or steel-cut oats, which are minimally processed, and sweetening them naturally with spices or fruits is a healthier choice.

- **Pasta made from Refined Grains:** Pasta made from refined wheat flour poses similar challenges as other refined grains, as it is quickly digested and can lead to significant blood sugar increases. Instead, choosing whole grain or whole wheat pasta, which is higher in fiber and nutrients, is a better option for those seeking to reverse T2D.

- **Pre-packaged Rice Mixes:** Pre-packaged rice mixes often contain high levels of sodium, artificial flavorings, and unnecessary additives, which can be detrimental for individuals managing T2D. These mixes not only contribute to high blood pressure but may also contain hidden sugars. Preparing brown rice or quinoa at home allows for better control over the ingredients and aligns with a healthier Reverse Type 2 Diabetes Diet.

* * *

In the subsequent section of this chapter, comprehensive tables are provided to outline foods that are non-compliant with Reverse Type 2 Diabetes Diet. These tables offer detailed information including serving size, Glycemic Index (GI), Glycemic Load (GL), and Net Carbohydrates for each food item. These metrics are particularly relevant when a food item's non-compliance is attributed to a high glycemic load and/or high carbohydrate content.

However, it is important to note that not all non-compliant foods can be categorized solely based on their GI, GL, or net carbohydrate content. Some food items are deemed non-compliant due to factors such as extensive processing, excessive sodium content, or an abundance of unhealthy fats. For these specific food items, detailed GI, GL, or net carb data may not be provided in the tables. Instead, they are simply listed with a note indicating their non-compliant status. This differentiation is aimed at ensuring clarity in understanding why certain food items are not recommended under the principles of the Reverse Type 2 Diabetes Diet.

GRAINS, CEREALS & PASTA

GRAINS, CEREALS & PASTA	SERVING SIZE	GI	GL	NET CARB
Barley Flour or Meal	½ cup, 64g	55	12	38g
Alpha-Bits	1 serving			
Apple Jacks	1 serving	Non-compliant foods		
Barley Malt Flour	½ cup, 61g	65	18	42g
Calrose Rice	½ cup cooked, 80g	75	27.5	37g
Canned Pasta Meals	1 serving	Non-compliant foods		
Cap'n Crunch	1 serving	Non-compliant foods		
Cereal Bars (different brands)	1 serving	Non-compliant foods		
Cinnamon Toast Crunch	1 cup, 31g	74	16	24g
Cinnamon Toast Crunch	1 serving	Non-compliant foods		
Cocoa Puffs	1 cup, 27g	77	23	24g
Cocoa Puffs	1 serving	Non-compliant foods		
Cookie Crisp	1 serving	Non-compliant foods		
Corn Flakes	1 cup, 28g	93	18	23g
Corn Flour Masa White	1 cup, 114g	60-65	42	77g
Corn Flour Whole-Grain Blue	1 cup, 128g	50-55	34	76g
Corn Flour Whole-Grain White	1 cup, 128g	50-55	34	76g
Corn Flour Whole-Grain Yellow	1 cup, 128g	50-55	34	76g
Corn Flour Yellow Degermed	1 cup, 125g	50-55	31	71g
Corn Pops	1 serving	Non-compliant foods		

GRAINS, CEREALS & PASTA	SERVING SIZE	GI	GL	NET CARB
Cornmeal Degermed White	1 cup, 138g	50-55	32	75g
Cornmeal Degermed White	1 cup, 138g	50-55	32	75g
Cornmeal Degermed Yellow	1 cup, 138g	50-55	32	75g
Cornstarch	1 cup, 128g	85-90	43	107g
Count Chocula	1 serving	Non-compliant foods		
Cream of Rice	1 cup cooked, 240g	70-85	20	27g
Cream of Wheat	1 cup cooked, 244g	70-85	19	26g
Farina	1 cup cooked, 242g	70-80	19	26g
Farro	1 cup cooked, 169g	40	18	45g
Froot Loops	1 cup, 29g	69	20	24g
Frosted Flakes	1 cup, 27g	55	16	26g
Frosted Flakes	1 serving	Non-compliant foods		
Fruit Loops	1 serving	Non-compliant foods		
Fruity Pebbles	1 serving	Non-compliant foods		
Garlic and Herb Penne	2 ounces, 56g	50	18	41g
Gluten Free Corn Noodles	1 cup, 200g	60-65	27	42g
Gluten-Free Penne	2 ounces, 56g	40	10	43g
Gluten-Free Spaghetti	1 cup cooked, 140g	52	24	46g
Glutinous Rice	1 cup cooked, 174g	86-91	37	42g
Golden Grahams	1 serving	Non-compliant foods		
Granola	1/2 cup, 61g	56-69	17	37g
Granola (different brands)	1 serving	Non-compliant foods		
Honey Smacks	1 serving	Non-compliant foods		
Instant Flavored Rice or Pasta Mixes	1 serving	Non-compliant foods		

GRAINS, CEREALS & PASTA	SERVING SIZE	GI	GL	NET CARB
Instant Oatmeal Packs (different brands)	1 serving	Non-compliant foods		
Lucky Charms	1 serving	Non-compliant foods		
Muesli with Added Sugars (different brands)	1 serving	Non-compliant foods		
Pop-Tarts Cereal	1 serving	Non-compliant foods		
Processed Bran Cereals (different brands)	1 serving	Non-compliant foods		
Puffed Rice or Corn Cereals (different brands)	1 serving	Non-compliant foods		
Reese's Puffs	1 serving	Non-compliant foods		
Rice Krispies Treats Cereal	1 serving	Non-compliant foods		
S'mores Cereal	1 serving	Non-compliant foods		
Seasoned Packaged Noodles	1 serving	Non-compliant foods		
Sugar-Sweetened Flakes (different brands)	1 serving	Non-compliant foods		
Sugary Cereals (different brands)	1 serving	Non-compliant foods		
Trix	1 serving	Non-compliant foods		

FISH, SEAFOOD, AND FISH PRODUCTS

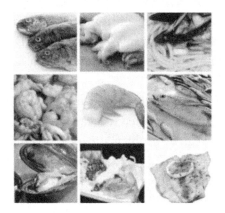

Fish and seafood are generally considered excellent sources of lean protein and omega-3 fatty acids, offering numerous health benefits and a low glycemic load (GL). However, some variations of these nutritious foods, due to their preparation or processing, may not align with a Type 2 Diabetes (T2D) reversal diet. High sodium content, heavy processing, breading, and certain cooking methods can transform these typically healthy options into potentially detrimental choices for individuals managing T2D and aiming for weight loss as per the twins cycle hypothesis.

Here are some categories that do not comply with the diet's principles:

- **Breaded and Fried Fish:** Although fish is naturally low in unhealthy fats and carbohydrates, when it's breaded and fried, it becomes a less healthy option. The breading, often composed of refined grains, introduces additional carbohydrates that can elevate blood sugar levels. Frying, on the other hand, can significantly increase calorie content and potentially foster insulin resistance. Therefore, it's better to avoid breaded and fried fish on a Reverse Type 2 Diabetes Diet.
- **Processed Seafood Products:** Items such as fish sticks, fish patties, and seafood nuggets often involve heavy processing and may contain additives, preservatives, and unhealthy fats. High in sodium, unhealthy oils, and even hidden sugars, these processed foods are not a smart choice for T2D management. Fresh or minimally processed seafood is a far healthier alternative.
- **Smoked and Cured Fish:** Smoked and cured fish products like smoked salmon or salted fish can have a high sodium content, which can be problematic for individuals with T2D. Excessive sodium intake can contribute to high blood pressure and increased cardiovascular risk. Consumption of these types of fish should be minimized, and lower-sodium alternatives should be considered instead.
- **Breaded and Fried Seafood:** Just like breaded and fried fish, breaded and fried seafood (such as shrimp or calamari) is high in unhealthy fats, calories, and refined grains. The breading and frying process can lead to blood sugar spikes and should be avoided on a Reverse Type 2 Diabetes Diet.
- **High Sodium Canned Fish:** Canned fish products, particularly those packed in brine or sauces, often contain excessive sodium, which can cause fluid retention and elevated blood pressure. Choosing low-sodium or no-salt-

added canned fish options can help minimize these negative effects.

Although fish and seafood provide numerous health benefits, it's crucial to make informed choices for a successful Reverse Type 2 Diabetes Diet. Avoid breaded and fried fish or seafood, heavily processed seafood products, smoked and cured fish, and high-sodium canned fish. Instead, prioritize fresh or minimally processed fish and seafood, and be mindful of cooking methods that minimize the addition of unhealthy fats, refined grains, and excessive sodium.

FRUITS AND FRUITS PRODUCTS

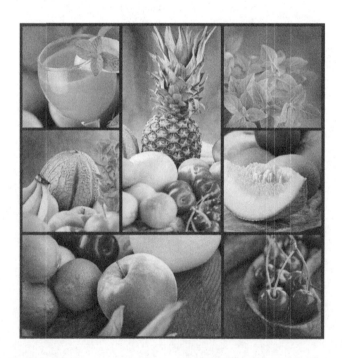

In the subsequent section of this chapter, comprehensive tables are provided to outline foods that are non-compliant with Reverse Type 2 Diabetes Diet. These tables offer detailed information including serving size, Glycemic Index (GI), Glycemic Load (GL), and Net Carbohydrates for each food item. These metrics are particularly relevant when a food item's non-compliance is attributed to a high glycemic load and/or high carbohydrate content.

However, it is important to note that not all non-compliant foods can be categorized solely based on their GI, GL, or net carbohydrate content. Some food items are deemed non-compliant due to factors such as extensive processing, excessive sodium content, or an abundance of unhealthy fats. For these specific food items, detailed GI, GL, or net carb data may not be provided in the tables. Instead, they are simply listed with a note indicating their non-compliant status. This differentiation is aimed at ensuring clarity in understanding why certain food items are not recommended under the principles of the Reverse Type 2 Diabetes Diet.

FRUITS & FRUIT PRODUCTS

FRUITS & FRUIT PRODUCTS	SERVING SIZE	GI	GL	NET CARB
Apple Candied	1 medium (60g)	High	High	Varies
Apple Fried	1 cup (124g)	Non-compliant foods		
Apple Jelly (store bought)	1 tbsp (20g)	High	High	Varies
Apple Rings Fried	1 cup (100g)	Non-compliant foods		
Apples (like in fried apple pies)	½ cup (59g)	Non-compliant foods		
Applesauce Canned Heavy Syrup Drained	1 tbsp (20g)	High	High	Varies
Applesauce Canned Sweetened	1 cup (250g)	High	High	43g
Apricot Dried Cooked With Sugar	1 cup (225g)	High	High	51g
Apricot Preserves (store bought)	1 tbsp (20g)	High	High	Varies
Apricots Canned Heavy Syrup Drained	1 cup (235g)	High	High	38g
Apricots Canned Heavy Syrup Drained	1 tbsp (20g)	High	High	Varies
Apricots Dehydrated Sulfured Stewed	1 cup (245g)	High	High	36g
Banana Batter-Dipped Fried	1 extra small (105g)	High	High	35g
Banana Red Fried	1 extra small (105g)	High	High	35g
Banana Ripe Fried	1 extra small (105g)	High	High	35g

FRUITS & FRUIT PRODUCTS	SERVING SIZE	GI	GL	NET CARB
Banana, ripe	1 extra small (105g)	85	26.5	31g
Banana, ripe Baked	1 extra small (105g)	High	High	28g
Bananas fritters	½ cup (59g)	Non-compliant foods		
Blackberries Canned Heavy Syrup Drained	1 cup (250g)	High	High	36g
Blackberries Canned Heavy Syrup Drained	1 tbsp (20g)	High	High	Varies
Blackberry Jam (store bought)	1 tbsp (20g)	High	High	Varies
Blueberries Canned Heavy Syrup	1 cup (256g)	High	High	33g
Blueberries Canned Heavy Syrup Drained	1 tbsp (20g)	High	High	Varies
Blueberry Jam (store bought)	1 tbsp (20g)	High	High	Varies
Boysenberries Canned Heavy Syrup	1 cup (250g)	High	High	36g
Boysenberries Canned Heavy Syrup Drained	1 tbsp (20g)	High	High	Varies
Cherry Jam (store bought)	1 tbsp (20g)	High	High	Varies
Cranberry Jelly (store bought)	1 tbsp (20g)	High	High	Varies
Cranberry sauce Canned Heavy Syrup Drained	1 tbsp (20g)	High	High	Varies
Cranberry sauce, Canned Heavy Syrup Drained	¼ cup (70g)	High	High	Varies
Dried Apricots, sweetened	¼ cup (32g)	High	High	Varies
Dried Banana, sweetened	¼ cup (30g)	High	High	Varies

FRUITS & FRUIT PRODUCTS	SERVING SIZE	GI	GL	NET CARB
Dried Blueberries, sweetened	¼ cup (40g)	High	High	Varies
Dried Cherries, sweetened	¼ cup (40g)	High	High	Varies
Dried Cranberries, sweetened	¼ cup (40g)	High	High	Varies
Dried Currants, sweetened	¼ cup (40g)	High	High	Varies
Dried Custard Apple Sweetened	¼ cup (30g)	High	High	Varies
Dried Kiwi, sweetened	¼ cup (30g)	High	High	Varies
Dried Longan	¼ cup (32g)	High	High	Varies
Dried Lychee, sweetened	¼ cup (30g)	High	High	Varies
Dried Mango, sweetened	¼ cup (30g)	High	High	Varies
Dried Papaya, sweetened	¼ cup (30g)	High	High	Varies
Dried Pear, sweetened	¼ cup (40g)	High	High	Varies
Dried Persimmon	¼ cup (32g)	High	High	Varies
Dried Persimmon, sweetened	¼ cup (32g)	High	High	Varies
Dried Pineapple Sweetened	¼ cup (40g)	High	High	Varies
Dried Pineapple, sweetened	¼ cup (35g)	High	High	Varies
Dried Sapodilla Sweetened	¼ cup (30g)	High	High	Varies
Fig Jam (store bought)	1 tbsp (20g)	High	High	Varies
Fried Apples	½ cup (59g)	Non-compliant foods		
Fried Mango	½ cup (59g)	Non-compliant foods		
Fried Peaches	½ cup (59g)	Non-compliant foods		
Fried pineapple fritters	½ cup (59g)	Non-compliant foods		

FRUITS & FRUIT PRODUCTS	SERVING SIZE	GI	GL	NET CARB
Fried Strawberries	½ cup (59g)	Non-compliant foods		
Golden Seedless Raisins	¼ cup (40g)	High	High	Varies
Grape Jelly (store bought)	1 tbsp (20g)	High	High	Varies
Grape Juice (store bought)	1 cup (253g)	High	High	Varies
Guava Nectar Canned	1 cup (240g)	High	High	Varies
Guava Nectar Canned Heavy Syrup Drained	1 tbsp (20g)	High	High	Varies
Kiwi Jam (store bought)	1 tbsp (20g)	High	High	Varies
Lemon Curd (store bought)	1 tbsp (20g)	High	High	Varies
Mango Jam (store bought)	1 tbsp (20g)	High	High	Varies
Mango Nectar Canned Heavy Syrup Drained	1 tbsp (20g)	High	High	Varies
Mixed Fruit Preserves (store bought)	1 tbsp (20g)	High	High	Varies
Nance Canned Heavy Syrup Drained	1 cup (160g)	High	High	Varies
Nance Canned Heavy Syrup Drained	1 tbsp (20g)	High	High	Varies
Orange Marmalade (store bought)	1 tbsp (20g)	High	High	Varies
Orange Pineapple Juice Blend (store bought)	1 cup (250g)	High	High	Varies
Peach Preserves (store bought)	1 tbsp (20g)	High	High	Varies
Peaches Spiced Canned Heavy Syrup	1 cup (250g)	High	High	Varies
Peaches Spiced Canned Heavy Syrup	1 tbsp (20g)	High	High	Varies

FRUITS & FRUIT PRODUCTS	SERVING SIZE	GI	GL	NET CARB
Pear Preserves (store bought)	1 tbsp (20g)	High	High	Varies
Pears Canned Heavy Syrup	1 cup (245g)	High	High	Varies
Pears Canned Heavy Syrup Drained	1 cup (242g)	High	High	Varies
Pears Canned Heavy Syrup Drained	1 tbsp (20g)	High	High	Varies
Pears Canned Heavy Syrup Drained	1 tbsp (20g)	High	High	Varies
Pineapple Canned Extra Heavy Syrup	1 cup (250g)	High	High	Varies
Pineapple Canned Extra Heavy Syrup	1 tbsp (20g)	High	High	Varies
Pineapple Canned Heavy Syrup	1 tbsp (20g)	High	High	Varies
Pineapple Canned Heavy Syrup Drained	1 cup (246g)	High	High	Varies
Pineapple Canned Heavy Syrup Drained	1 cup (248g)	High	High	Varies
Pineapple Canned Heavy Syrup Drained	1 tbsp (20g)	High	High	Varies
Pineapple Canned Heavy Syrup Drained	1 tbsp (20g)	High	High	Varies
Pineapple Frozen Chunks Sweetened	1 cup (165g)	58	24.3	42g
Pineapple Jam (store bought)	1 tbsp (20g)	High	High	Varies
Pineapple, Canned Heavy Syrup Drained	½ cup (122g)	High	High	Varies
Plantains Cooked	½ cup mashed (100g)	55	17.6	32g
Plantains fried	½ cup (59g)	Non-compliant foods		
Plantains Green Fried	½ cup (59g)	Non-compliant foods		

FRUITS & FRUIT PRODUCTS	SERVING SIZE	GI	GL	NET CARB
Plum Jam (store bought)	1 tbsp (20g)	High	High	Varies
Plums Canned Heavy Syrup Drained	½ cup (125g)	High	High	Varies
Plums Canned Heavy Syrup Drained	1 tbsp (20g)	High	High	Varies
Raisin	¼ cup (40g)	66	20.5	31g
Raspberry Jam (store bought)	1 tbsp (20g)	High	High	Varies
Strawberry Jam (store bought)	1 tbsp (20g)	High	High	Varies
Sweetened Dried Apples	¼ cup (35g)	High	High	Varies
Sweetened Dried Blueberries	¼ cup (35g)	High	High	Varies
Sweetened Dried Cherries	¼ cup (40g)	High	High	Varies
Sweetened Dried Cranberries	¼ cup (40g)	High	High	Varies
Sweetened Dried Mango	¼ cup (40g)	High	High	Varies
Sweetened Dried Peaches	¼ cup (38g)	High	High	Varies
Sweetened Dried Pears	¼ cup (40g)	High	High	Varies
Sweetened Dried Plums	¼ cup (40g)	High	High	Varies
Watermelon Jelly (store bought)	1 tbsp (20g)	High	High	Varies

MEATS - BEEF, LAMP, VEAL, PORK & POULTRY

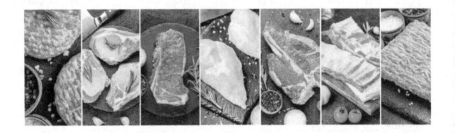

Here are some categories that do not comply with the diet's principles.

SAUSAGES AND SIMILAR PROCESSED MEATS

Sausages and similar processed meats encompass a diverse range of products such as andouille sausage, bacon, bratwurst, chorizo, hot dogs, salami, and many more.

Non-Compliance with Reverse Type 2 Diabetes Diet: These types of foods often do not conform to the principles of the Reverse Type 2 Diabetes Diet or the 2020-2025 Dietary Guidelines for Americans (DGA).

Processed meats like sausages typically contain high amounts of sodium and can also be rich in saturated fats, both of which can contribute to elevated blood pressure and cardiovascular disease risk - two health aspects that people with diabetes need to closely manage.

Added to this, processed meats may include additives such as nitrates and nitrites, which have been linked to a range of health issues. Moreover, the protein content in these foods can also be problematic for those with diabetes and Chronic Kidney Disease (CKD), as overconsumption of protein can strain the kidneys.

In terms of carbohydrates, some sausages and similar processed meats may contain fillers or flavorings that increase their sugar content, potentially leading to unpredictable effects on blood glucose levels.

Furthermore, these foods typically lack dietary fiber, an essential nutrient for regulating blood sugar levels and promoting overall digestive health.

Given their high sodium content, potential sugar content, lack of fiber, and potential health risks associated with certain additives, sausages and similar processed meats are generally not recommended for those seeking to manage or reverse T2D. When making food choices, always scrutinize nutrition labels and aim to select fresh, minimally processed foods wherever possible.

🚫 *Andouille sausage* 🚫 *Bacon* 🚫 *BBQ sausage rolls* 🚫 *Beef sausage rolls* 🚫 *Black forest ham* 🚫 *Black forest ham slices* 🚫 *Black pudding* 🚫 *Blood sausage* 🚫 *Bockwurst* 🚫 *Bologna* 🚫 *Bratwurst* 🚫 *Breakfast sausage links* 🚫 *Breakfast sausage rolls* 🚫 *Cajun-style sausage* 🚫 *Cajun-style sausage (full-fat)* 🚫 *Capicola* 🚫 *Capicola slices* 🚫 *Cervelat* 🚫 *Cheese and sausage rolls* 🚫 *Chicken sausage rolls* 🚫 *Chicken sausages (commercially made)* 🚫 *Chorizo* 🚫 *Chorizo sausage rolls* 🚫 *Classic pork sausage rolls* 🚫 *Corned beef* 🚫 *Corned venison* 🚫 *Cured duck breast* 🚫 *Deviled ham* 🚫 *Duck confit* ⊘ *Finnish sausage* ⊘ *Frankfurters* ⊘ *Genoa salami* ⊘ *Goetta* ⊘ *Ham (commercially made)* ⊘ *Head cheese* ⊘ *Honey-baked turkey (commercially made)* ⊘ *Honey-glazed ham (commercially made)* ⊘ *Honey-roasted ham (commercially made)* ⊘ *Honey-smoked turkey (commercially made)* ⊘ *Hot dogs* ⊘ *Italian salami (full-fat)* ⊘ *Italian sausage* ⊘ *Italian sausage (regular)* ⊘ *Kabanosy* ⊘ *Kielbasa* ⊘ *Lebanon bologna* ⊘ *Linguica* ⊘ *Liverwurst* ⊘ *Lunch meats (e.g., turkey, chicken, roast beef)* ⊘ *Merguez sausage* ⊘ *Mortadella* ⊘ *Mortadella slices* ⊘ *Pastrami slices* ⊘ *Peppered salami* ⊘ *Pepperoni* ⊘ *Pickled pork* ⊘ *Polish sausage* ⊘ *Potted meat* ⊘ *Prosciutto slices* ⊘ *Salami* ⊘ *Sausages* ⊘ *Smoked beef brisket* ⊘ *Smoked beef ribs* ⊘ *Smoked ham hock slices* ⊘ *Smoked ham shank slices* ⊘ *Smoked ham shoulder slices* ⊘ *Smoked ham slices* ⊘ *Smoked ham steak slices* ⊘ *Smoked pork ribs* ⊘ *Smoked sausages (full-fat)* ⊘ *Smoked turkey/chicken breast* ⊘ *Soppressata* ⊘ *South African boerewors* ⊘ *Summer sausage* ⊘ *Thuringer sausage* ⊘ *Turkey bacon* ⊘ *Turkey pastrami* ⊘ *Turkey roll* ⊘ *Turkey sausage rolls* ⊘ *Turkey sausages (commercially made)* ⊘ *Vienna sausages* ⊘ *Vienna sausages (full-fat)* ⊘ *Weisswurst* ⊘ *White pudding*

BREADED AND DEEP-FRIED/BREADED AND FRIED FOODS

Breaded and deep-fried or simply fried foods include a wide variety of items such as breaded and fried cutlets of various meats, breaded and deep-fried chicken bites, and similar items.

Non-Compliance with Reverse Type 2 Diabetes Diet: These foods typically do not align well with the principles of the Reverse Type 2 Diabetes Diet or the 2020-2025 Dietary Guidelines for Americans

(DGA). They are often highly processed, high in unhealthy fats, and contain significant amounts of simple carbohydrates.

Breaded and fried foods are often high in trans and saturated fats due to the frying process. These fats can heighten the risk of heart disease, which individuals with diabetes are already at a higher risk of. Furthermore, the breading on these foods often contains refined flours with a high glycemic index (GI) that can lead to rapid spikes in blood sugar levels.

Moreover, these foods can be high in sodium, which can negatively impact blood pressure and cardiovascular health. The protein content in some of these foods can also pose a problem for individuals with diabetes and Chronic Kidney Disease (CKD) as excessive protein can strain the kidneys.

Additionally, breaded and fried foods often lack dietary fiber, which is essential for maintaining stable blood sugar levels and promoting overall digestive health.

Given their high GI, unhealthy fat content, and potential lack of key nutrients, breaded and deep-fried or fried foods are typically not the best choice for individuals trying to reverse T2D. As with any food choices, reading nutrition labels and prioritizing whole, unprocessed foods can make a significant difference in managing and improving health outcomes.

> ⊘ *Breaded and deep-fried chicken bites* ⊘ *Breaded and deep-fried chicken breasts* ⊘ *Breaded and deep-fried chicken chunks* ⊘ *Breaded and deep-fried chicken cutlets* ⊘ *Breaded and deep-fried chicken dippers* ⊘ *Breaded and deep-fried chicken drumsticks* ⊘ *Breaded and deep-fried chicken escalopes* ⊘ *Breaded and deep-fried chicken fillets* ⊘ *Breaded and deep-fried chicken fingers* ⊘ *Breaded and deep-fried chicken fritters* ⊘ *Breaded and deep-fried chicken goujons* ⊘ *Breaded and deep-fried chicken lollipops* ⊘ *Breaded and deep-fried chicken*

nuggets Ⓢ *Breaded and deep-fried chicken patties* Ⓢ
Breaded and deep-fried chicken popcorn Ⓢ *Breaded and
deep-fried chicken strips* Ⓢ *Breaded and deep-fried
chicken tenders* Ⓢ *Breaded and deep-fried chicken thighs*
Ⓢ *Breaded and deep-fried chicken wings* Ⓢ *Breaded and
fried beef cutlets* Ⓢ *Breaded and fried cauliflower cutlets*
Ⓢ *Breaded and fried chicken cutlets* Ⓢ *Breaded and fried
chicken schnitzel* Ⓢ *Breaded and fried clam cutlets* Ⓢ
Breaded and fried crab cutlets Ⓢ *Breaded and fried
eggplant cutlets* Ⓢ *Breaded and fried fish cutlets* Ⓢ
Breaded and fried lamb cutlets Ⓢ *Breaded and fried
lobster cutlets* Ⓢ *Breaded and fried mushroom cutlets* Ⓢ
Breaded and fried oyster cutlets Ⓢ *Breaded and fried pork
cutlets* Ⓢ *Breaded and fried pork schnitzel* Ⓢ *Breaded
and fried potato cutlets* Ⓢ *Breaded and fried scallop
cutlets* Ⓢ *Breaded and fried seitan cutlets* Ⓢ *Breaded and
fried shrimp cutlets* Ⓢ *Breaded and fried tempeh cutlets*
Ⓢ *Breaded and fried tofu cutlets* Ⓢ *Breaded and fried
turkey cutlets* Ⓢ *Breaded and fried turkey schnitzel* Ⓢ
Breaded and fried veal cutlets Ⓢ *Breaded and fried veal
schnitzel* Ⓢ *Breaded and fried zucchini cutlets* Ⓢ
Breaded calamari rings Ⓢ *Breaded clams* Ⓢ *Breaded
crab cakes* Ⓢ *Breaded crab sticks* Ⓢ *Breaded fish cakes*
Ⓢ *Breaded fish fillets* Ⓢ *Breaded fish fingers* Ⓢ *Breaded
fish nuggets* Ⓢ *Breaded fish sandwiches* Ⓢ *Breaded fish
sandwiches* Ⓢ *Breaded fish sticks* Ⓢ *Breaded lobster bites*
Ⓢ *Breaded lobster bites* Ⓢ *Breaded oysters* Ⓢ *Breaded
oysters* Ⓢ *Breaded scallops* Ⓢ *Breaded scallops* Ⓢ
Breaded shrimp Ⓢ *Tempura-battered calamari* Ⓢ
Tempura-battered clams Ⓢ *Tempura-battered crab sticks*
Ⓢ *Tempura-battered fish* Ⓢ *Tempura-battered oysters* Ⓢ
Tempura-battered scallops Ⓢ *Tempura-battered
shrimp*

SLICED MEATS

Sliced meats, often used for sandwiches, include a variety of cold cuts, such as roast beef slices, ham slices, turkey slices, and other similar products.

Non-Compliance with Reverse Type 2 Diabetes Diet: According to the principles of the Reverse Type 2 Diabetes Diet and the 2020-2025 Dietary Guidelines for Americans (DGA), sliced meats for sandwiches are generally discouraged. These products are typically processed, can contain high levels of sodium, and may include additives and preservatives.

Sliced meats' high sodium content can have detrimental effects on blood pressure and overall cardiovascular health, which is especially crucial for individuals with diabetes. In addition, the protein content in sliced meats could pose challenges for individuals managing T2D and Chronic Kidney Disease (CKD), as excessive protein consumption can overtax the kidneys.

Problematic Pairing with Bread: Sliced meats are often paired with bread to make sandwiches. However, many types of bread have a high Glycemic Index (GI), meaning they can rapidly raise blood sugar levels. This combination can be particularly problematic for individuals with T2D, as it can lead to increased carbohydrate intake and difficulty controlling blood sugar levels.

Furthermore, sliced meats and bread both typically lack significant amounts of dietary fiber. Fiber is essential for blood sugar regulation and digestive health, emphasizing these foods' unsuitability in a diet aimed at reversing T2D.

While sliced meats can provide convenience, individuals aiming for T2D reversal should carefully consider their health impacts. Reading nutritional labels, making mindful dietary choices, and opting for whole, unprocessed foods whenever possible are vital steps in maintaining a balanced, health-promoting diet.

Ⓢ Roast beef slices Ⓢ Turkey breast slices Ⓢ Ham slices Ⓢ Chicken breast slices Ⓢ Pastrami slices Ⓢ Corned beef slices Ⓢ Salami slices Ⓢ Pepperoni slices Ⓢ Prosciutto slices Ⓢ Mortadella slices Ⓢ Genoa salami slices Ⓢ Capicola slices Ⓢ Bologna slices Ⓢ Smoked turkey breast slices Ⓢ Smoked ham slices Ⓢ Smoked chicken breast slices Ⓢ Smoked salmon slices Ⓢ Smoked roast beef slices Ⓢ Smoked turkey/chicken breast slices Ⓢ Black forest ham slices Ⓢ Honey-roasted ham slices Ⓢ Honey-baked turkey slices Ⓢ Turkey pastrami slices Ⓢ Smoked bacon slices Ⓢ Roast lamb slices Ⓢ Roast pork slices Ⓢ Roast chicken slices Ⓢ Turkey pastrami slices Ⓢ Smoked chicken slices Ⓢ Smoked turkey slices Ⓢ Black forest ham slices Ⓢ Honey-roasted ham slices Ⓢ Roast lamb slices Ⓢ Roast pork slices Ⓢ Roast chicken slices Ⓢ Smoked bacon slices Ⓢ Turkey bacon slices Ⓢ Pancetta slices Ⓢ Canadian bacon slices Ⓢ Roast beef slices (seasoned/flavored variations) Ⓢ Turkey breast slices (seasoned/flavored variations) Ⓢ Ham slices (seasoned/flavored variations) Ⓢ Chicken breast slices (seasoned/flavored variations) Ⓢ Pastrami slices (seasoned/flavored variations) Ⓢ Corned beef slices (seasoned/flavored variations) Ⓢ Salami slices (seasoned/flavored variations) Ⓢ Pepperoni slices (seasoned/flavored variations) Ⓢ Prosciutto slices (seasoned/flavored variations) Ⓢ Mortadella slices (seasoned/flavored variations) Ⓢ Genoa salami slices (seasoned/flavored variations) Ⓢ Capicola slices (seasoned/flavored variations) Ⓢ Bologna slices (seasoned/flavored variations)

CANNED/PRESERVED MEATS:

Canned or preserved meats are products that have undergone preservation methods such as canning, curing, or drying to extend their shelf life and make them more convenient for storage and use. Examples include canned corned beef, canned roast beef, canned ham, canned pork, and other similar products.

Non-Compliance with Reverse Type 2 Diabetes Diet: As per the principles of the Reverse Type 2 Diabetes Diet and the 2020-2025 Dietary Guidelines for Americans (DGA), the consumption of canned or preserved meats is generally not recommended. These products tend to be heavily processed, contain high levels of sodium, and often incorporate additives and preservatives.

Canned or preserved meats' high sodium content can negatively affect blood pressure and overall cardiovascular health, significant considerations for individuals with diabetes. Moreover, their protein content, while potentially beneficial in moderation, can be problematic for those managing T2D alongside Chronic Kidney Disease (CKD), as overconsumption of protein can put stress on the kidneys.

Additionally, some preserved meats may contain added sugars, which can contribute to higher carbohydrate intake and impact blood sugar levels. Pairing these meats with high Glycemic Index (GI) foods can lead to rapid increases in blood sugar levels, adding to the difficulty of effective T2D management.

Lastly, these products are typically low in dietary fiber, a crucial nutrient for blood sugar regulation and overall digestive health. This further limits their suitability in a diet aimed at reversing T2D.

Therefore, while canned and preserved meats may offer convenience, individuals aiming for T2D reversal should carefully consider their potential health impacts. Reading nutritional labels attentively and making mindful dietary choices are vital steps towards maintaining a balanced, healthful diet.

Canned anchovies in oil Ⓢ *Canned bacon* Ⓢ *Canned barbecue pork* Ⓢ *Canned beef chili* Ⓢ *Canned beef chunks* Ⓢ *Canned beef gravy* Ⓢ *Canned beef gravy mix*

⊘ Canned beef in BBQ sauce ⊘ Canned beef in gravy
⊘ Canned beef pot roast ⊘ Canned beef pot roast with
vegetables ⊘ Canned beef ravioli ⊘ Canned beef ravioli
in tomato sauce ⊘ Canned beef stew ⊘ Canned beef stew
with vegetables ⊘ Canned beef stroganoff ⊘ Canned
beef tamales ⊘ Canned chicken ⊘ Canned chicken
alfredo ⊘ Canned chicken and dumplings ⊘ Canned
chicken and rice soup ⊘ Canned chicken chunks ⊘
Canned chicken curry ⊘ Canned chicken gravy ⊘
Canned chicken gravy mix ⊘ Canned chicken in
barbecue sauce ⊘ Canned chicken in cream sauce ⊘
Canned chicken noodle soup ⊘ Canned chicken pot pie
⊘ Canned chicken salad ⊘ Canned chicken spread ⊘
Canned chicken tamales ⊘ Canned chicken tikka masala
⊘ Canned chili con carne ⊘ Canned corned beef ⊘
Canned corned beef hash ⊘ Canned corned beef spread
⊘ Canned corned mutton ⊘ Canned deviled ham ⊘
Canned duck confit ⊘ Canned ham ⊘ Canned ham
slices ⊘ Canned ham spread ⊘ Canned hot dogs ⊘
Canned liver pâté ⊘ Canned luncheon meat ⊘ Canned
meat chili ⊘ Canned meat curry ⊘ Canned meat pies
⊘ Canned meat sauce ⊘ Canned meat tamales ⊘
Canned meat tortellini ⊘ Canned meat-based pasta sauce
⊘ Canned meatballs ⊘ Canned meatballs in sauce ⊘
Canned meatloaf ⊘ Canned mixed meat stew ⊘ Canned
pork ⊘ Canned pork and beans ⊘ Canned pork in gravy
⊘ Canned pork shoulder ⊘ Canned pork spread ⊘
Canned potted meat ⊘ Canned pulled pork ⊘ Canned
roast beef ⊘ Canned roast beef slices ⊘ Canned sausages
in tomato sauce ⊘ Canned spam ⊘ Canned turkey ⊘
Canned turkey breast slices ⊘ Canned turkey chili ⊘
Canned turkey chili with beans ⊘ Canned turkey gravy
⊘ Canned turkey gravy mix ⊘ Canned turkey meatballs
⊘ Canned turkey pot pie ⊘ Canned turkey spread ⊘
Canned Vienna sausages

SMOKED MEATS

Smoked meats include a variety of animal-based products, ranging from pork and beef to seafood such as catfish and clams. The smoking process, which involves curing the meat with smoke from burning or smoldering materials like wood, gives these products a distinctive flavor.

Non-Compliance with Reverse Type 2 Diabetes Diet: The principles of the Reverse Type 2 Diabetes Diet, guided by the 2020-2025 Dietary Guidelines for Americans (DGA), typically discourage the consumption of smoked meats. These meats are processed and often high in sodium and additives, which could pose challenges for blood sugar management and overall health.

Though smoked meats may be an appealing choice for their distinct taste, their high sodium content can negatively impact blood pressure and cardiovascular health, both significant considerations for individuals with diabetes. Moreover, smoked meats, like any protein-rich food, consumed in large quantities can pose challenges for individuals managing diabetes alongside Chronic Kidney Disease (CKD). Over-consumption of protein can put stress on the kidneys and exacerbate CKD.

In addition, pairing smoked meats with high Glycemic Index (GI) foods can lead to sharp rises in blood glucose levels, presenting an additional concern for people with diabetes. High GI foods cause an abrupt spike in blood sugar levels, which can make it challenging to manage diabetes effectively.

It's essential for individuals aiming to manage or reverse T2D to carefully consider the potential impacts of their food choices on their health. This involves being mindful of nutritional labels and being cautious about pairing high sodium or protein foods with high GI foods. Despite the flavor appeal of smoked meats, their nutritional profile may make them less suitable for a diet aimed at T2D reversal.

🚫 Smoked andouille sausage 🚫 Smoked bacon 🚫 Smoked beef brisket 🚫 Smoked beef jerky 🚫 Smoked beef ribs 🚫 Smoked beef sausage 🚫 Smoked beef tenderloin 🚫 Smoked beef tri-tip 🚫 Smoked bison ribs 🚫 Smoked bison sausage 🚫 Smoked bologna 🚫 Smoked bratwurst 🚫 Smoked chicken 🚫 Smoked chicken breast 🚫 Smoked chicken drumsticks 🚫 Smoked chicken sausage 🚫 Smoked chicken thighs 🚫 Smoked chicken wings 🚫 Smoked chorizo 🚫 Smoked corned beef 🚫 Smoked duck breast 🚫 Smoked duck legs 🚫 Smoked elk sausage 🚫 Smoked elk tenderloin 🚫 Smoked goat chops 🚫 Smoked goat sausage 🚫 Smoked goat shoulder 🚫 Smoked goose breast 🚫 Smoked ham 🚫 Smoked ham hock 🚫 Smoked ham shank 🚫 Smoked ham slices 🚫 Smoked ham steak 🚫 Smoked hot dogs 🚫 Smoked kangaroo steak 🚫 Smoked lamb chops 🚫 Smoked lamb leg 🚫 Smoked lamb shoulder 🚫 Smoked ostrich fillets 🚫 Smoked pastrami 🚫 Smoked pepperoni 🚫 Smoked pheasant 🚫 Smoked pork 🚫 Smoked pork belly 🚫 Smoked pork chops 🚫 Smoked pork sausage 🚫 Smoked pork shoulder 🚫 Smoked pork tenderloin 🚫 Smoked pulled pork 🚫 Smoked quail 🚫 Smoked rabbit 🚫 Smoked salami 🚫 Smoked sausage (e.g., smoked kielbasa, smoked bratwurst) 🚫 Smoked sausage links (e.g., smoked breakfast sausage links) 🚫 Smoked sausage patties (e.g., smoked breakfast sausage patties) 🚫 Smoked turkey 🚫 Smoked turkey bacon 🚫 Smoked turkey breast 🚫 Smoked turkey legs 🚫 Smoked turkey sausage 🚫 Smoked turkey wings 🚫 Smoked venison jerky 🚫 Smoked venison sausage 🚫 Smoked venison tenderloin 🚫 Smoked wild boar ribs 🚫 Smoked wild boar sausage 🚫 Smoked wild boar shoulder

COMMERCIALLY MADE/PROCESSED POULTRY

Commercially made or processed poultry items refer to chicken, turkey, and other poultry products that are mass-produced. These products, such as chicken nuggets, chicken patties, chicken tenders, and honey-baked turkey, often contain additives and preservatives and tend to be high in sodium.

Non-Compliance with Reverse Type 2 Diabetes Diet: Consistent with 2020-2025 Dietary Guidelines for Americans (DGA) and principles of the Reverse Type 2 Diabetes Diet, commercially processed poultry products are generally not advised. These items are often prepared with unhealthy cooking methods, like deep-frying, and contain unhealthy additives that may hinder blood sugar management and overall health.

While commercially processed poultry products are quick and convenient, they pose potential health risks. Their high sodium content can negatively affect blood pressure and cardiovascular health, which is already a concern for those with diabetes. Moreover, these products often have added sugars, unhealthy fats, and other additives that can contribute to blood sugar fluctuations.

Additionally, for those managing diabetes along with Chronic Kidney Disease (CKD), consuming these high-protein foods in large amounts can strain the kidneys, potentially worsening CKD.

Therefore, despite their convenience, commercially processed poultry products may not be an optimal choice for individuals aiming to manage or reverse T2D, especially those with additional health considerations like CKD. It's always prudent to review nutritional labels carefully and to consider the potential health impacts before integrating such foods into one's diet.

Breaded chicken bites ⊘ Breaded chicken burgers ⊘
Breaded chicken cutlets ⊘ Breaded chicken dippers ⊘
Breaded chicken drumsticks ⊘ Breaded chicken fillets ⊘

Breaded chicken fingers Ⓢ *Breaded chicken meatballs* Ⓢ
Breaded chicken popcorn Ⓢ *Breaded chicken schnitzel* Ⓢ
Breaded chicken strips Ⓢ *Breaded chicken wings* Ⓢ
Chicken nuggets Ⓢ *Chicken patties* Ⓢ *Chicken tenders*
Ⓢ *Grilled chicken breast strips* Ⓢ *Grilled chicken patties*
Ⓢ *Grilled chicken tenders* Ⓢ *Grilled turkey breast slices*
Ⓢ *Grilled turkey deli meat* Ⓢ *Honey-baked turkey* Ⓢ
Honey-glazed turkey Ⓢ *Honey-roasted turkey* Ⓢ
Honey-smoked turkey Ⓢ *Processed chicken burger patties*
Ⓢ *Processed chicken deli meats (e.g., chicken ham)* Ⓢ
Processed chicken lunch meats (e.g., chicken bologna) Ⓢ
Processed chicken meatballs Ⓢ *Processed chicken*
sausages (e.g., chicken hot dogs) Ⓢ *Processed turkey deli*
meats (e.g., turkey ham) Ⓢ *Processed turkey lunch meats*
(e.g., turkey bologna) Ⓢ *Processed turkey meatballs* Ⓢ
Processed turkey sausages (e.g., turkey hot dogs) Ⓢ
Roasted chicken breast Ⓢ *Roasted chicken slices* Ⓢ
Roasted turkey breast Ⓢ *Roasted turkey slices* Ⓢ *Smoked*
turkey breast Ⓢ *Smoked turkey deli meat* Ⓢ *Smoked*
turkey slices

PIES AND SIMILAR

Pies and similar products are prepared by filling a pastry crust with a variety of ingredients, then baking the mixture until it's ready to serve. This category includes an array of dishes like chicken and mushroom pies, chicken pot pies, cottage pie, curry meat pies, lamb meat pies, shepherd's pie, steak and kidney pies, tourtière, turkey pot pies, and vegetable and meat pies.

Non-Compliance with Reverse Type 2 Diabetes Diet: According to 2020-2025 Dietary Guidelines for Americans (DGA) and the principles of the Reverse Type 2 Diabetes Diet, foods like pies are typically not recommended. They are often made with refined flour and contain additives that may interfere with blood sugar management and overall health. Furthermore, the filling may have high levels of fat and salt, and sometimes even added sugars.

While pies may seem like a comforting meal option, their high carbo-hydrate content from the pastry crust, potential for added sugars, and high fat content can pose challenges for individuals with diabetes. This is especially the case for those also dealing with CKD, as the high protein content in meat-based pies can put additional strain on already compromised kidneys.

Thus, despite their convenience and taste appeal, pies may not be the best choice for individuals trying to manage or reverse T2D, particu-larly those with additional health concerns like CKD. As always, it's advisable to read nutritional labels carefully and to take potential health impacts into account before incorporating such foods into one's diet.

Beef and ale pies ⊘ Beef and Guinness pies ⊘ Beef and mushroom pies ⊘ Beef and onion pies ⊘ Beef and Stilton pies ⊘ Beef and vegetable pies ⊘ Chicken and asparagus pies ⊘ Chicken and bacon pies ⊘ Chicken and chorizo pies ⊘ Chicken and ham pies ⊘ Chicken and leek pies ⊘ Chicken and mushroom pies ⊘ Chicken and spinach pies ⊘ Chicken and sweetcorn pies ⊘ Chicken and vegetable pies ⊘ Chicken pot pies ⊘ Cottage pie ⊘ Curry meat pies ⊘ Lamb and mint pies ⊘ Lamb and potato pies ⊘ Lamb and rosemary pies ⊘ Lamb and vegetable pies ⊘ Lamb meat pies ⊘ Mushroom and leek pies ⊘ Mushroom and Stilton pies ⊘ Mushroom and tarragon pies ⊘ Pork and apple pies ⊘ Pork and black pudding pies ⊘ Pork and sage pies ⊘ Shepherd's pie ⊘ Spinach and feta pies ⊘ Spinach and mushroom pies ⊘ Steak and kidney pies ⊘ Tourtière ⊘ Turkey and cranberry pies ⊘ Turkey and ham pies ⊘ Turkey and stuffing pies ⊘ Turkey pot pies ⊘ Vegetable and meat pies ⊘ *Vegetarian pies (e.g., vegetable pie, cheese and onion pie)*

JERKIES

Jerky is lean meat that has been trimmed of fat, cut into strips, and then dried to prevent spoilage. Usually, this drying includes the addition of salt to prevent bacteria from developing on the meat before sufficient moisture has been removed.

Non-Compliance with Reverse Type 2 Diabetes Diet: As per the 2020-2025 Dietary Guidelines for Americans (DGA) and the principles of Type 2 Diabetes (T2D) reversal diet, processed foods like jerky are generally not recommended. They often lack key nutrients and contain additives that can interfere with blood sugar management and overall health.

Thus, while jerky might seem like a convenient source of protein, its high sodium and protein content, along with potential added sugars and lack of fiber, make it less suitable for people with diabetes, particularly those also dealing with CKD. Always read the nutritional labels carefully and consider the potential impacts on your health before including it in your diet.

⊘ *Alligator jerky* ⊘ *BBQ pork jerky* ⊘ *Beef jerky* ⊘ *Bison jerky* ⊘ *Cajun-style alligator jerky* ⊘ *Carolina Reaper hot pepper beef jerky* ⊘ *Chicken jerky* ⊘ *Chicken teriyaki jerky* ⊘ *Chipotle pork jerky* ⊘ *Citrus teriyaki salmon jerky* ⊘ *Cranberry maple elk jerky* ⊘ *Elk jerky* ⊘ *Garlic and black pepper beef jerky* ⊘ *Hickory-smoked venison jerky* ⊘ *Honey mustard chicken jerky* ⊘ *Honey sriracha buffalo jerky* ⊘ *Honey-glazed turkey jerky* ⊘ *Kangaroo jerky* ⊘ *Lemon pepper turkey jerky* ⊘ *Maple brown sugar bacon jerky* ⊘ *Maple-glazed bacon jerky* ⊘ *Ostrich jerky* ⊘ *Peppered beef jerky* ⊘ *Peppered venison jerky* ⊘ *Pork jerky* ⊘ *Salmon jerky* ⊘ *Sesame ginger turkey jerky* ⊘ *Smoked salmon jerky* ⊘ *Smoky barbecue bison jerky* ⊘ *Smoky mesquite trout jerky* ⊘ *Spicy buffalo jerky* ⊘ *Sriracha chicken jerky* ⊘ *Sweet and spicy jerky* ⊘ *Sweet mesquite pork jerky* ⊘ *Teriyaki kangaroo jerky* ⊘ *Teriyaki venison jerky* ⊘ *Trout jerky* ⊘ *Tuna jerky* ⊘ *Turkey jerky* ⊘ *Venison jerky*

High Fat Ground Meats

High fat ground meats include products such as fatty ground turkey, ground lamb with a higher fat percentage, ground pork with a higher fat percentage, and ground veal with a higher fat percentage.

Non-Compliance with Reverse Type 2 Diabetes Diet: Ground meats with high fat content are typically not recommended as per the 2020-2025 Dietary Guidelines for Americans (DGA) and the principles of the Reverse Type 2 Diabetes Diet.

Highly fatty meats, particularly when they are processed or cooked in unhealthy ways, can lead to excessive intake of saturated fats. This can contribute to higher cholesterol levels, increased risk of heart disease, and weight gain, all of which are health concerns for individuals managing diabetes.

Moreover, the protein content of these ground meats can also be problematic for those with diabetes and Chronic Kidney Disease (CKD), as excessive protein consumption can exacerbate kidney function issues.

The fact that these are ground meats also often means they've been mechanically processed, which can sometimes involve the use of additives and preservatives that aren't conducive to a Reverse Type 2 Diabetes Diet.

These meats generally lack fiber and can be paired with high Glycemic Index (GL) foods, such as bread or pasta, leading to potential spikes in blood sugar levels.

Thus, high fat ground meats can pose various challenges in the management and potential reversal of T2D. Whenever possible, choose lean cuts of fresh meat over high-fat or processed options, and consider pairing them with low GL foods for optimal blood glucose control.

- ⊘ *Ground beef (regular or high-fat)* ⊘ *Ground pork* ⊘ *Ground lamb* ⊘ *Ground veal* ⊘ *Ground duck* ⊘ *Ground goose* ⊘ *Ground bison* ⊘ *Ground sausage (various flavors)*
- ⊘ *Ground chorizo* ⊘ *Ground fatty cuts of beef, such as chuck or brisket (when ground)* ⊘ *Ground fatty cuts of pork, such as shoulder or belly (when ground)* ⊘ *Ground fatty cuts of lamb, such as shoulder or leg (when ground)* ⊘ *Ground fatty cuts of veal, such as shoulder or rib (when ground)* ⊘ *Ground fatty cuts of duck, such as leg or breast (when ground)* ⊘ *Ground fatty cuts of goose, such as leg or breast (when ground)* ⊘ *Ground fatty cuts of bison, such as chuck or rib (when ground)* ⊘ *Ground fatty cuts of turkey, such as thigh or dark meat (when ground)* ⊘ *Ground fatty cuts of chicken, such as thigh or dark meat (when ground)* ⊘ *Ground fatty cuts of game meats, such as venison or wild boar (when ground)* ⊘ *Ground fatty cuts of other animal meats, such as rabbit or kangaroo (when ground)*

OTHER PROCESSED MEATS

"Other Processed Meats" is a category that encompasses a variety of meat products, including Black pudding, Blood sausage, Corned beef, Corned venison, Duck confit, Head cheese, Liverwurst, etc.

Non-Compliance with Reverse Type 2 Diabetes Diet: The 2020-2025 Dietary Guidelines for Americans (DGA) and the principles of the

Reverse Type 2 Diabetes Diet discourage the consumption of highly processed meats.

These kinds of processed meats often contain additives, preservatives, and are typically high in sodium, all of which can negatively impact blood sugar management and overall health in people with diabetes.

Similar to other processed meats, these products can also be high in fat and protein. Excessive intake of fats, particularly saturated and trans fats, can contribute to elevated cholesterol levels, and increased risk of heart disease. On the other hand, excessive protein can be a concern for individuals with diabetes and Chronic Kidney Disease (CKD), as it can exacerbate kidney function issues.

These meats also tend to lack fiber, a key nutrient that can help regulate blood sugar levels and support overall digestive health.

Additionally, these types of processed meats are often consumed in combination with high Glycemic Index (GL) foods, which can lead to sudden spikes in blood sugar levels.

Therefore, while these "other processed meats" might be appealing for their unique flavors and convenience, their potential negative health impacts make them less suitable for those seeking to manage or reverse T2D. Instead, focus on fresh, minimally processed meats and pair them with low GL foods for better blood glucose control.

> Ⓢ *Black pudding* Ⓢ *Blood sausage* Ⓢ *Corned beef* Ⓢ
> *Corned venison* Ⓢ *Duck confit* Ⓢ *Head cheese* Ⓢ
> *Liverwurst* Ⓢ *Mortadella* Ⓢ *Pancetta* Ⓢ *Pastrami* Ⓢ
> *Pepperoni* Ⓢ *Prosciutto* Ⓢ *Salami Milano* Ⓢ *Salami*
> *Genoa*Ⓢ *Salami Soppressata* Ⓢ *Sausage Italian* Ⓢ
> *Sausage bratwurst* Ⓢ *Vienna sausage*

NUTS AND SEEDS

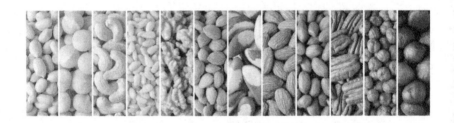

Here are some categories that do not comply with the diet's principles.

HONEY-ROASTED OR SUGARED NUTS

Nuts are generally a nutritious snack option, packed with beneficial fats, protein, and fiber. However, when they're honey-roasted or coated with sugar, they become far less suitable for individuals following a Type 2 Diabetes (T2D) reversal diet.

Non-Compliance with Reverse Type 2 Diabetes Diet: Honey-roasted or sugared nuts typically don't align with the principles of the Reverse

Type 2 Diabetes Diet and the 2020-2025 Dietary Guidelines for Americans (DGA).

When nuts are honey-roasted or coated with sugar, their carbohydrate and sugar content experiences a significant increase. These additional sugars can cause a rapid surge in blood sugar levels, which poses a challenge for individuals with diabetes or those aiming to reverse T2D.

Moreover, the roasting procedure may involve the use of unhealthy oils, resulting in an elevated intake of unhealthy fats. Consuming excessive amounts of unhealthy fats can contribute to weight gain and other health illnesses, including heart disease.

Furthermore, the added sugars and flavors can make these nuts more palatable and potentially lead to overeating, which can further contribute to weight gain – a factor that can worsen insulin resistance and hinder the process of reversing T2D.

Given their high sugar content and the potential for overeating, honey-roasted or sugared nuts are typically not the best choice for individuals managing or trying to reverse T2D. Opt instead for unsweetened, raw, or dry-roasted nuts, which provide the nutritional benefits of nuts without the added sugars. Always remember to pay attention to portion sizes, as even the healthiest of nuts are calorie-dense.

⊘ *Candied almonds* ⊘ *Candied cashews* ⊘ *Candied peanuts* ⊘ *Candied pecans* ⊘ *Candied pistachios* ⊘ *Candied walnuts* ⊘ *Frosted almonds* ⊘ *Frosted cashews* ⊘ *Frosted peanuts* ⊘ *Frosted pecans* ⊘ *Frosted pistachios* ⊘ *Frosted walnuts* ⊘ *Glazed almonds* ⊘ *Glazed cashews* ⊘ *Glazed peanuts* ⊘ *Glazed pecans* ⊘ *Glazed pistachios* ⊘ *Glazed walnuts* ⊘ *Honey-roasted almonds* ⊘ *Honey-roasted cashews* ⊘ *Honey-roasted peanuts* ⊘ *Honey-roasted pecans* ⊘ *Honey-roasted pistachios* ⊘ *Honey-roasted walnuts* ⊘ *Sugared almonds*

⊘ *Sugared cashews* ⊘ *Sugared peanuts* ⊘ *Sugared pecans* ⊘ *Sugared pistachios* ⊘ *Sugared walnuts*

SWEETENED NUT BUTTERS

While nut butters can be a good source of healthy fats and protein, those that have added sugars or sweeteners can contribute to elevated blood sugar levels, making them less suitable for individuals following a Type 2 Diabetes (T2D) reversal diet.

Non-Compliance with Reverse Type 2 Diabetes Diet: Sweetened nut butters often conflict with the principles of the Reverse Type 2 Diabetes Diet and the 2020-2025 Dietary Guidelines for Americans (DGA).

Nut butters (e.g., peanut butter, almond butter, cashew butter) can be part of a healthy diet due to their high protein and healthy fat content. However, when sweeteners or sugars are added, these otherwise healthy options can become problematic for individuals managing or reversing T2D. The added sugars increase the overall carbohydrate content, potentially causing spikes in blood sugar levels.

These products can also contribute to weight gain when consumed in excess, particularly because the added sweetness can make them easy to overeat. Weight management is crucial for those with T2D, as it can directly impact insulin sensitivity and overall blood glucose control.

Furthermore, sweetened nut butters often contain unhealthy oils and additives, detracting from their nutritional benefits.

Given the potential negative effects on blood sugar control and weight management, sweetened nut butters are not the best choice for those seeking to manage or reverse T2D. It's recommended to opt for natural, unsweetened varieties of nut butters and pay close attention to portion sizes due to their raised calorie content.

⊘ Brownie batter peanut butter ⊘ Butter toffee almond butter ⊘ Cherry almond butter ⊘ Chocolate banana hazelnut spread ⊘ Chocolate chip cookie dough peanut butter ⊘ Chocolate mint cashew butter ⊘ Chocolate coconut almond butter ⊘ Chocolate hazelnut spread ⊘ Cinnamon raisin peanut butter ⊘ ⊘ Cinnamon swirl peanut butter ⊘ Coconut maple pecan butter ⊘ Cookie butter spread ⊘ Espresso almond butter ⊘ Gingerbread spice almond butter ⊘ Graham cracker almond butter ⊘ Honey roasted cashew butter ⊘ Honey-flavored peanut butter ⊘ Honey roasted walnut butter ⊘ Maple pecan almond butter ⊘ Maple-flavored almond butter ⊘ Marshmallow-flavored peanut butter ⊘ Mocha hazelnut spread ⊘ Mocha-flavored almond butter ⊘ Peppermint chocolate hazelnut spread ⊘ Pumpkin spice almond butter ⊘ Salted caramel peanut butter ⊘ Salted caramel pecan butter ⊘ Salted caramel macadamia nut butter ⊘ Salted toffee peanut butter ⊘ Strawberry shortcake almond butter ⊘ Snickerdoodle cashew butter ⊘ Sweetened cinnamon almond butter ⊘ Vanilla chai cashew butter ⊘ Vanilla-flavored cashew butter ⊘ White chocolate macadamia nut butter

SUGARED OR GLAZED SEEDS

While seeds are generally a good source of healthy fats, fiber, and essential nutrients, when they're coated with sugar or a glaze, their carbohydrate and added sugar content can rise significantly, making them less appropriate for individuals following a Type 2 Diabetes (T2D) reversal diet.

Non-Compliance with Reverse Type 2 Diabetes Diet: Sugared or glazed seeds often conflict with the principles of the Reverse Type 2 Diabetes Diet and the 2020-2025 Dietary Guidelines for Americans (DGA).

Seeds, such as pumpkin, sunflower, or flax seeds, naturally have a balanced profile of protein, healthy fats, and fiber, which aids in blood sugar regulation. However, the addition of a sugary coating increases their carbohydrate content, potentially leading to spikes in blood sugar levels.

Moreover, sugared or glazed seeds can contribute to weight gain if consumed excessively due to their elevated calorie content. Weight management is crucial in controlling and reversing T2D because it directly influences insulin sensitivity and overall glucose management.

In addition to sugar, these products may contain unhealthy oils and additives, which further decrease their nutritional value.

Due to their potential impact on blood sugar control and weight management, sugared or glazed seeds aren't the most beneficial option for those aiming to manage or reverse T2D. Instead, it's advised to select plain seeds and to be aware of portion sizes due to their high calorie content.

> ⊘ *Candied sunflower seeds* ⊘ *Caramel-covered pepitas (pumpkin seeds)* ⊘ *Caramelized pepitas (pumpkin seeds)* ⊘ *Chocolate-covered flaxseeds* ⊘ *Cinnamon-glazed sunflower kernels* ⊘ *Cinnamon-sugar coated sesame seeds* ⊘ *Coconut-coated chia seeds* ⊘ *Frosted flaxseeds* ⊘ *Frosted hemp seeds* ⊘ *Glazed sesame seeds* ⊘ *Honey-coated flaxseeds* ⊘ *Honey-glazed pumpkin seeds* ⊘ *Honey-roasted sunflower kernels* ⊘ *Honeyed poppy seeds* ⊘ *Maple-coated sesame seeds* ⊘ *Maple-flavored poppy seeds* ⊘ *Sugared pumpkin seeds* ⊘ *Sugared sunflower kernels* ⊘ *Sweetened chia seeds* ⊘ *Sweetened hemp seeds*

OIL AND CONDIMENTS

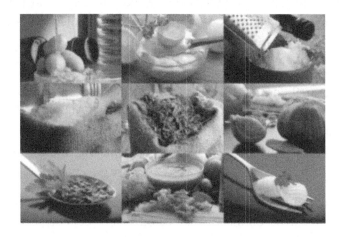

Effective management and reversal of Type 2 Diabetes (T2D) necessitate a comprehensive and nuanced approach to dietary choices. This doesn't merely involve the total quantity of fats and oils consumed, but also encapsulates the quality of those fats, their sources, and the cooking techniques employed. Certain oils, fats, and condiments have properties that can exert a negative influence on blood sugar levels, weight control, and overall health. Understanding these intricacies is vital in the journey towards T2D reversal.

NON-COMPLIANT OILS AND FATS:

Palm and Coconut oils, along with Lard, are high in saturated fats. Regular consumption of these can negatively affect cholesterol levels, insulin sensitivity, and increase the risk of heart disease. Vegetable shortening and some margarine products contain trans fats, which have been directly linked to heart disease.

Grapeseed and Cottonseed oils, rich in polyunsaturated fats, contain a high omega-6 fatty acid content. The disproportionate ratio of omega-6 to omega-3 fatty acids can result in inflammation, which poses a risk factor for chronic conditions like T2D. Processed foods such as pastries and snacks often contain hydrogenated or partially hydrogenated oils, which harbor detrimental trans fats.

Animal-based fats, especially those derived from red and processed meats, have elevated levels of saturated fats and cholesterol. Fat drippings from processed meats like sausages or bacon are also high in unhealthy fats.

Cooking methods matter too. Deep frying can contribute to the creation of Advanced Glycation End-products (AGEs), which have been linked to chronic ailments (e.g, diabetes and heart disease). Also, frying oils can surpass their smoke point, making the oil toxic and harmful to health.

Switching to oils high in monounsaturated and polyunsaturated fats, like olive oil, avocado oil, and canola oil, can be beneficial. These oils align with the principles of the Reverse Type 2 Diabetes Diet, contributing to improved heart health.

Remember, while fats are an essential part of our diet, it's the type of fat that matters. Prioritize unsaturated fats over saturated and trans fats, consider the smoke point when cooking, and monitor the ratio of omega-6 to omega-3 fatty acids in your diet.

NON-COMPLIANT CONDIMENTS:

Many condiments, despite being used in small quantities, can be high in sugars, unhealthy fats, or sodium, which may not align with Reverse Type 2 Diabetes Diet.

Examples of such condiments include:

- Ketchup, barbecue sauce, and sweet chili sauce, which often contain high amounts of added sugars.
- Mayonnaise and some salad dressings, high in unhealthy fats.
- Soy sauce, pickles, and other pickled or brined condiments, which can contain high levels of sodium.
- Teriyaki sauce: Teriyaki sauce often contains a significant amount of added sugars, which can negatively impact blood sugar levels. Look for low-sugar or sugar-free alternatives.
- Sweet and sour sauce: Similar to teriyaki sauce, sweet and sour sauce is typically high in added sugars. Choose options with reduced or no sugar.
- Honey mustard: While mustard itself is generally a healthier choice, honey mustard often contains added sugars. Opt for regular mustard or make your own sugar-free version.
- Barbecue and marinade sauces: Many barbecue and marinade sauces are loaded with sugar and can contribute to elevated blood sugar levels. Look for low-sugar or sugar-free options, or consider making your own using natural sweeteners in moderation.
- Syrups and toppings: Maple syrup, chocolate syrup, and other dessert toppings are high in sugars. Avoid or limit their use in your Reverse Type 2 Diabetes Diet.
- Relish: Some commercial relish products can contain added sugars and high amounts of sodium. Choose sugar-free or homemade relish options.

Remember to carefully read food labels when purchasing condiments, as ingredients and nutritional content can vary among brands. Opting for homemade versions or using herbs, spices, and vinegar-based dressings can help you avoid unnecessary sugars, unhealthy fats, and excessive sodium.

MEDITERRANEAN RESTAURANT FOODS

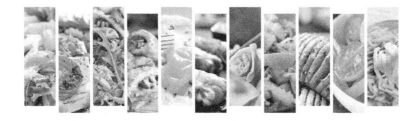

While the Mediterranean Diet (MedDiet) is praised for its health-promoting qualities, especially its benefits for heart health and blood sugar regulation, not all foods served in Mediterranean restaurants align with Reverse Type 2 Diabetes Diet. This diet combines the principles of the Glycemic Load (GL) framework, elements of the MedDiet, weight management strategies, caloric restriction, and the 2020-2025 General Dietary Advices (GDAs). The following food categories and items typically found in Mediterranean restaurants may not be compliant with Reverse Type 2 Diabetes Diet.

HIGH GLYCEMIC LOAD FOODS:

Even within the MedDiet, there are foods with high Glycemic Load, which can cause blood sugar spikes. These include refined breads and pastries often served in restaurants, such as pita bread, baklava, and other sweet pastries. Also, dishes that are primarily based on white rice or pasta can have a high GL. Examples of such foods include:

     ⊘ *Alcoholic beverages with added sugars (e.g., sweet wines, fruity cocktails)* ⊘ *Baklava* ⊘ *Basbousa* ⊘ *Couscous-based dishes* ⊘ *Dessert crepes with sweet fillings* ⊘ *Dishes with sugary glazes or sauces (e.g., honey-glazed chicken)* ⊘ *Ekmek Kataifi* ⊘ *Fruit-based desserts with added sugars (e.g., fruit tarts, fruit crumbles)* ⊘ *Galaktoboureko* ⊘ *Gullac* ⊘ *Halva* ⊘ *High-sugar fruit preserves used in dishes or as toppings* ⊘ *High-sugar fruit sorbets or gelatos* ⊘ *Kanafeh* ⊘ *Kataifi* ⊘ *Kazandibi* ⊘ *Lokma* ⊘ *Loukoumades* ⊘ *Mahalabiya* ⊘ *Malabi* ⊘ *Pastries or desserts made with refined flour and high sugar content* ⊘ *Pizza with a refined white flour crust* ⊘ *Potato-based dishes (e.g., fried potatoes, potato salads)* ⊘ *Ravani* ⊘ *Rice pudding or other sweet rice-based desserts* ⊘ *Saragli* ⊘ *Şekerpare* ⊘ *Stuffed grape leaves (dolmades) made with white rice* ⊘ *Sutlac (Rice Pudding)* ⊘ *Sweetened baklava or other pastries with high sugar content* ⊘ *Sweetened coffee beverages (e.g., flavored lattes, caramel macchiatos)* ⊘ *Sweetened fruit cocktails or punches* ⊘ *Sweetened tea or iced tea* ⊘ *Sweetened yogurt desserts (e.g., Greek yogurt with added sugars)* ⊘ *Tavuk Göğsü* ⊘ *Tulumba* ⊘ *White pasta dishes* ⊘ *White pita bread* ⊘ *White rice pilaf*

DEEP-FRIED FOODS:

Despite the MedDiet's overall focus on healthy fats, Mediterranean restaurants may serve deep-fried foods such as falafel, fried calamari, or French fries. These foods can be high in unhealthy fats and calories, which can contribute to weight gain and hinder T2D reversal. Examples of such foods include:

◎ *Arancini (fried rice balls)* ◎ *Berenjenas con miel (fried eggplant with honey)* ◎ *Bourekas (fried stuffed pastries)* ◎ *Churros (fried dough pastry)* ◎ *Falafel* ◎ *Fried anchovies* ◎ *Fried artichokes* ◎ *Fried beef kofta (Kofta fritte)* ◎ *Fried calamari* ◎ *Fried calamari rings (Calamari fritti)* ◎ *Fried capers* ◎ *Fried chicken (Pollo fritto)* ◎ *Fried dough balls (Struffoli)* ◎ *Fried dough puffs (Zeppole fritte)* ◎ *Fried dough strips (Sfinci di San Giuseppe)* ◎ *Fried doughnuts (Bomboloni)* ◎ *Fried eggplant* ◎ *Fried eggs* ◎ *Fried falafel balls (Falafel fritti)* ◎ *Fried feta cheese (Feta fritta)* ◎ *Fried fish (Pesce fritto)* ◎ *Fried halloumi cheese (Halloumi fritto)* ◎ *Fried lamb chops (Cotolette d'agnello fritte)* ◎ *Fried mussels (Cozze fritte)* ◎ *Fried olives* ◎ *Fried onion* ◎ *Fried sardines* ◎ *Fried shellfish* ◎ *Fried shrimp (Gamberi fritti)* ◎ *Fried veal cutlets (Cotolette di vitello fritte)* ◎ *Fried zucchini* ◎ *Frittelle (fried sweet fritters)* ◎ *Keftedes (fried meatballs)* ◎ *Loukoumades (fried doughnuts)* ◎ *Panelle (fried chickpea fritters)* ◎ *Pastilla (fried Moroccan pastry)* ◎ *Patatas bravas (fried potatoes with sauce)* ◎ *Patates tiyanites (fried potatoes)* ◎ *Pimientos de Padrón (fried Padrón peppers)* ◎ *Saganaki (fried cheese)*

HIGH-SODIUM FOODS:

While the traditional MedDiet is low in sodium, restaurant versions of Mediterranean dishes can be quite high in salt. Dishes like moussaka, gyro, and certain types of cheese (like halloumi or feta) can have a high sodium content, which is not suitable for a Reverse Type 2 Diabetes Diet focused on maintaining healthy blood pressure levels.

Ⓢ *Anchovy paste* Ⓢ *Anchovy-based sauces or dressings (e.g., bagna cauda, boquerones)* Ⓢ *Bottarga (salted, cured fish roe)* Ⓢ *Bouillabaisse (traditional Mediterranean fish stew)* Ⓢ *Bruschetta with salted or marinated toppings* Ⓢ *Canned fish in brine or saltwater* Ⓢ *Capers (often pickled in salt)* Ⓢ *Cured olives* Ⓢ *Dolmades (stuffed grape leaves)* Ⓢ *Feta cheese* Ⓢ *Fish soups or chowders* Ⓢ *Graviera cheese (a Greek cheese with a salty flavor)* Ⓢ *Gyro (grilled meat typically served in a pita bread)* Ⓢ *Halloumi cheese* Ⓢ *Kalamata olives (marinated in brine)* Ⓢ *Marinated feta cheese (often preserved in a salty brine)* Ⓢ *Marinated mushrooms with added salt* Ⓢ *Marinated or salted octopus* Ⓢ *Moussaka (layers of eggplant, ground meat, and béchamel sauce)* Ⓢ *Olives marinated in brine or saltwater* Ⓢ *Pecorino Romano cheese (a salty Italian cheese)* Ⓢ *Salted anchovies* Ⓢ *Salted cod (Bacalhau)* Ⓢ *Salted crackers or breadsticks* Ⓢ *Salted cured ham (e.g., Prosciutto, Jamón serrano)* Ⓢ *Salted cured meats (e.g., Salami, Chorizo)* Ⓢ *Salted fish (e.g., Salted mackerel, Salted herring)* Ⓢ *Salted nuts or nut mixes* Ⓢ *Salted or brined anchovy fillets* Ⓢ *Salted or brined cured hams (e.g., Prosciutto, Jamón serrano)* Ⓢ *Salted or marinated artichokes* Ⓢ *Salted or pickled vegetables (e.g., pickled eggplant, pickled peppers)* Ⓢ *Salted sardines* Ⓢ *Salted vegetables (e.g., pickled cucumbers, pickled cabbage)* Ⓢ *Sardine pâté or spread* Ⓢ *Spanakopita (spinach and feta pastry)* Ⓢ *Tapenade (olive-based spread)* Ⓢ *Taramasalata (fish roe dip)* Ⓢ *Tiropita (cheese pastry)* Ⓢ *Tzatziki sauce (yogurt and cucumber dip)*

HIGH-FAT MEATS:

Some Mediterranean restaurant dishes may include high-fat meats, such as lamb or certain cuts of beef. While the MedDiet encourages lean proteins, these high-fat meats can lead to increased caloric intake and hinder weight management, thus not aligning with Reverse Type 2 Diabetes Diet.

> Ⓢ *Beef Brisket* Ⓢ *Beef Burgers (made with higher fat content)* Ⓢ *Beef Ribeye Steak (Bistecca alla fiorentina)* Ⓢ *Beef Salami* Ⓢ *Beef Short Ribs* Ⓢ *Beef T-bone Steak (Bistecca alla fiorentina)* Ⓢ *Chicken Drumsticks (with skin)* Ⓢ *Chicken Liver Pâté* Ⓢ *Chicken Sausages (higher fat content)* Ⓢ *Chicken Thighs (with skin)* Ⓢ *Chicken Wings (with skin)* Ⓢ *Duck Breast* Ⓢ *Duck Confit (Confit de canard)* Ⓢ *Foie gras* Ⓢ *Lamb Kebabs (Shish kebabs)* Ⓢ *Lamb Kofta* Ⓢ *Lamb Shanks* Ⓢ *Lamb Shoulder* Ⓢ *Merguez Sausages* Ⓢ *Pork Belly* Ⓢ *Pork Chops* Ⓢ *Pork Ribs* Ⓢ *Pork Salami* Ⓢ *Pork Sausages* Ⓢ *Sausages made with higher fat content (e.g., lamb sausages, beef sausages, and chorizo)*

SUGARY BEVERAGES AND DESSERTS:

Traditional Mediterranean desserts and sweetened beverages served in restaurants, such as baklava, galaktoboureko, sweetened Greek coffee, or sweetened iced tea, can be high in added sugars, leading to blood sugar spikes and weight gain.

> Ⓢ *Greek Baklava Ice Cream* Ⓢ *Greek Galaktoboureko (phyllo pastry with sweet semolina custard filling)* Ⓢ *Greek Kourabiedes (almond butter cookies)* Ⓢ *Greek Loukoumades (honey-soaked fried dough balls)* Ⓢ *Greek Melomakarona (honey-soaked spice cookies)* Ⓢ *Greek Revani (syrup-soaked semolina cake)* Ⓢ *Italian Cannoli*

Siciliani (fried pastry tubes filled with sweet ricotta) Ⓢ
Italian Gelato (traditional Italian ice cream) Ⓢ *Italian
Granita (flavored crushed ice)* Ⓢ *Italian Panettone (sweet
bread loaf with dried fruits)* Ⓢ *Italian Panna Cotta
(cooked cream dessert)* Ⓢ *Italian Tiramisu (coffee-soaked
sponge cake layered with mascarpone cream)* Ⓢ *Italian
Zeppole (fried dough balls dusted with powdered sugar)* Ⓢ
*Lebanese Atayef (stuffed pancakes with sweet cheese or
nuts)* Ⓢ *Lebanese Ayran (a yogurt-based drink sweetened
with sugar)* Ⓢ *Lebanese Mafroukeh (sweet pistachio and
semolina dessert)* Ⓢ *Lebanese Mhalabiyeh (milk pudding
flavored with rosewater or orange blossom water)* Ⓢ
*Lebanese Osmalieh (shredded phyllo pastry with sweet
cream filling)* Ⓢ *Moroccan Bastilla (sweet and savory
layered pie)* Ⓢ *Moroccan Chebakia (honey-coated sesame
cookies)* Ⓢ *Moroccan Honey-Sweetened Pastries (e.g.,
msemen, shebakia)* Ⓢ *Moroccan Makrout (deep-fried
semolina cookies with date filling)* Ⓢ *Moroccan Mint Tea
with Sugar* Ⓢ *Moroccan Orange Blossom Water Pudding
(Mahalabiya)* Ⓢ *Moroccan Sellou (sweet sesame and
almond-based treat)* Ⓢ *Portuguese Pasteis de Nata
(custard tarts)* Ⓢ *Sicilian Cannoli (fried pastry tubes filled
with sweet ricotta cheese)* Ⓢ *Spanish Churros (fried dough
sticks coated in sugar)* Ⓢ *Spanish Flan (caramel custard)*
Ⓢ *Spanish Horchata* Ⓢ *Spanish Leche Frita (fried milk
pudding)* Ⓢ *Spanish Polvorones (crumbly almond cookies)*
Ⓢ *Spanish Torrijas (sweet soaked bread similar to French
toast)* Ⓢ *Traditional Greek Frappé* Ⓢ *Turkish Baklava
(layers of filo pastry with sweet syrup and nuts)* Ⓢ
Turkish Delight (gelatinous sweet confectionery) Ⓢ
Turkish Kazandibi (caramelized milk pudding) Ⓢ *Turkish
Lokma (fried dough balls soaked in syrup)* Ⓢ *Turkish
Sütlaç (rice pudding)* Ⓢ *Turkish Tea with Sugar (Çay)*

* * *

In the subsequent section of this chapter, comprehensive tables are provided to outline foods that are non-compliant with Reverse Type 2 Diabetes Diet. These tables offer detailed information including serving size, Glycemic Index (GI), Glycemic Load (GL), and Net Carbohydrates for each food item. These metrics are particularly relevant when a food item's non-compliance is attributed to a high glycemic load and/or high carbohydrate content.

However, it is important to note that not all non-compliant foods can be categorized solely based on their GI, GL, or net carbohydrate content. Some food items are deemed non-compliant due to factors such as extensive processing, excessive sodium content, or an abundance of unhealthy fats. For these specific food items, detailed GI, GL, or net carb data may not be provided in the tables. Instead, they are simply listed with a note indicating their non-compliant status. This differentiation is aimed at ensuring clarity in understanding why certain food items are not recommended under the principles of the Reverse Type 2 Diabetes Diet.

VEGETABLES AND VEGETABLE PRODUCTS

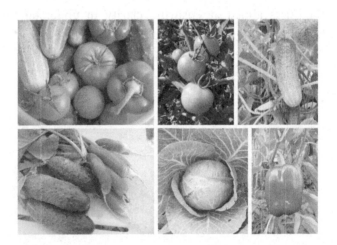

In the subsequent section of this chapter, comprehensive tables are provided to outline foods that are non-compliant with Reverse Type 2 Diabetes Diet. These tables offer detailed information including serving size, Glycemic Index (GI), Glycemic Load (GL), and Net Carbohydrates for each food item. These metrics are particularly relevant when a food item's non-compliance is attributed to a high glycemic load and/or high carbohydrate content.

However, it is important to note that not all non-compliant foods can be categorized solely based on their GI, GL, or net carbohydrate content. Some food items are deemed non-compliant due to factors such as extensive processing, excessive sodium content, or an abundance of unhealthy fats. For these specific food items, detailed GI, GL, or net carb data may not be provided in the tables. Instead, they are simply listed with a note indicating their non-compliant status. This differentiation is aimed at ensuring clarity in understanding why certain food items are not recommended under the principles of the Reverse Type 2 Diabetes Diet.

VEGETABLES & VEGETABLE PRODUCTS

VEGETABLES & VEGETABLE PRODUCTS	SERVING SIZE	GI	GL	NET CARB
Asparagus Chips, commercially made	1 oz (28g)	Non-compliant Foods		
Balsamic Glazed Grilled Red Onions	½ cup (115 g)	High	High	Varies
Beets Chips, commercially made	1 oz (28g)	Non-compliant Foods		
Bell peppers (red, yellow, or green) Chips, commercially made	1 oz (28g)	Non-compliant Foods		
Broccoli with Cheese Sauce	½ cup (115 g)	Non-compliant Foods		
Brussels sprouts Chips, commercially made	1 oz (28g)	Non-compliant Foods		
Butternut squash Chips, commercially made	1 oz (28g)	Non-compliant Foods		
Candied Sweet Potatoes	½ cup (115 g)	High	High	Varies
Carrots Chips, commercially made	1 oz (28g)	Non-compliant Foods		
Cauliflower in Cheese Sauce	½ cup (115 g)	Non-compliant Foods		
Celeriac (celery root) Chips, commercially made	1 oz (28g)	Non-compliant Foods		
Celery Chips, commercially made	1 oz (28g)	Non-compliant Foods		
Chard Chips, commercially made	1 oz (28g)	Non-compliant Foods		
Corn Casserole	½ cup (115 g)	Non-compliant Foods		
Corn on the cob with butter and/or sugar	½ cup (115 g)	Non-compliant Foods		
Creamed Corn	½ cup (115 g)	Non-compliant Foods		

VEGETABLES & VEGETABLE PRODUCTS	SERVING SIZE	GI	GL	NET CARB
Creamed Spinach	½ cup (115 g)	Non-compliant Foods		
Creamy Asparagus	½ cup (115 g)	Non-compliant Foods		
Creamy Coleslaw	½ cup (115 g)	Non-compliant Foods		
Creamy Corn	½ cup (115 g)	Non-compliant Foods		
Creamy Potato Salad	½ cup (115 g)	Non-compliant Foods		
Cucumbers Chips, commercially made	1 oz (28g)	Non-compliant Foods		
Eggplant Chips, commercially made	1 oz (28g)	Non-compliant Foods		
French Fries	½ cup (115 g)	High	High	Varies
Fried Artichoke Hearts	½ cup (115 g)	Non-compliant Foods		
Fried Asparagus	½ cup (115 g)	Non-compliant Foods		
Fried Avocado Slices	½ cup (115 g)	Non-compliant Foods		
Fried Broccoli	½ cup (115 g)	Non-compliant Foods		
Fried Brussels Sprouts	½ cup (115 g)	Non-compliant Foods		
Fried Cauliflower	½ cup (115 g)	Non-compliant Foods		
Fried Corn Nuggets	½ cup (115 g)	Non-compliant Foods		
Fried Eggplant	½ cup (115 g)	Non-compliant Foods		
Fried Green Beans	½ cup (115 g)	Non-compliant Foods		
Fried Green Tomatoes	½ cup (115 g)	Non-compliant Foods		
Fried Jalapeno Poppers	½ cup (115 g)	Non-compliant Foods		
Fried Mushrooms	½ cup (115 g)	Non-compliant Foods		
Fried Okra	½ cup (115 g)	Non-compliant Foods		
Fried Pickles	½ cup (115 g)	Non-compliant Foods		
Fried Plantains	½ cup (115 g)	Non-compliant Foods		
Fried Sweet Potato Fries	½ cup (115 g)	Non-compliant Foods		
Fried Tofu	½ cup (115 g)	Non-compliant Foods		

VEGETABLES & VEGETABLE PRODUCTS	SERVING SIZE	GI	GL	NET CARB
Fried Zucchini	½ cup (115 g)	Non-compliant Foods		
General Tso's Vegetables	½ cup (115 g)	Non-compliant Foods		
Glazed Carrots	½ cup (115 g)	Non-compliant Foods		
Green Bean Casserole	½ cup (115 g)	Non-compliant Foods		
Green beans Chips, commercially made	1 oz (28g)	Non-compliant Foods		
Grilled Lemon-Honey Glazed Zucchini	½ cup (115 g)	Non-compliant Foods		
Grilled Pineapple with Brown Sugar Glaze	½ cup (115 g)	Non-compliant Foods		
Grilled Soy-Ginger Glazed Eggplant	½ cup (115 g)	Non-compliant Foods		
Grilled Sweet and Spicy Glazed Corn on the Cob	½ cup (115 g)	Non-compliant Foods		
Grilled Sweet Chili Glazed Bell Peppers	½ cup (115 g)	Non-compliant Foods		
Grilled Teriyaki Glazed Vegetables	½ cup (115 g)	Non-compliant Foods		
Grilled vegetables with a high-sugar glaze or marinade	½ cup (115 g)	Non-compliant Foods		
Honey-Glazed Brussels Sprouts	½ cup (115 g)	Non-compliant Foods		
Honey-Glazed Grilled Carrots	½ cup (115 g)	Non-compliant Foods		
Jerusalem artichoke Chips, commercially made	1 oz (28g)	Non-compliant Foods		
Jicama Chips, commercially made	1 oz (28g)	Non-compliant Foods		
Kale Chips, commercially made	1 oz (28g)	Non-compliant Foods		
Kung Pao Vegetables	½ cup (115 g)	Non-compliant Foods		
Lotus root Chips, commercially made	1 oz (28g)	Non-compliant Foods		

VEGETABLES & VEGETABLE PRODUCTS	SERVING SIZE	GI	GL	NET CARB
Maple-Glazed Grilled Sweet Potatoes	½ cup (115 g)	Non-compliant Foods		
Mashed Potatoes with heavy cream and butter	½ cup (115 g)	Non-compliant Foods		
Okra Chips, commercially made	1 oz (28g)	Non-compliant Foods		
Onion Rings	½ cup (115 g)	Non-compliant Foods		
Orange-Glazed Grilled Brussels Sprouts	½ cup (115 g)	Non-compliant Foods		
Parsnips Chips, commercially made	1 oz (28g)	Non-compliant Foods		
Peas and Carrots with added sugar	½ cup (115 g)	Non-compliant Foods		
Plantains Chips, commercially made	1 oz (28g)	Non-compliant Foods		
Potato Gratin with cream and cheese	½ cup (115 g)	Non-compliant Foods		
Potato Pancakes	½ cup (115 g)	Non-compliant Foods		
Potatoes Au Gratin	½ cup (115 g)	Non-compliant Foods		
Pumpkin Chips, commercially made	1 oz (28g)	Non-compliant Foods		
Radishes Chips, commercially made	1 oz (28g)	Non-compliant Foods		
Rutabaga Chips, commercially made	1 oz (28g)	Non-compliant Foods		
Scalloped Potatoes	½ cup (115 g)	Non-compliant Foods		
Snow peas Chips, commercially made	1 oz (28g)	Non-compliant Foods		
Spinach Chips, commercially made	1 oz (28g)	Non-compliant Foods		
Sweet and Sour Cabbage	½ cup (115 g)	Non-compliant Foods		
Sweet and Sour Vegetables	½ cup (115 g)	Non-compliant Foods		

VEGETABLES & VEGETABLE PRODUCTS	SERVING SIZE	GI	GL	NET CARB
Sweet Chili Vegetable Stir-fry	½ cup (115 g)	Non-compliant Foods		
Sweet Glazed Carrots	½ cup (115 g)	Non-compliant Foods		
Sweet Maple Glazed Beets	½ cup (115 g)	Non-compliant Foods		
Sweet Potato Casserole with marshmallows and brown sugar	½ cup (115 g)	Non-compliant Foods		
Sweet potatoes Chips, commercially made	1 oz (28g)	Non-compliant Foods		
Szechuan Vegetables	½ cup (105g)	Non-compliant Foods		
Tempura Vegetables	½ cup (115 g)	Non-compliant Foods		
Teriyaki Vegetables	½ cup (115 g)	Non-compliant Foods		
Turnips Chips, commercially made	1 oz (28g)	Non-compliant Foods		
Vegetable Chow Mein	½ cup (115 g)	Non-compliant Foods		
Vegetable Fried Rice	½ cup (115 g)	Non-compliant Foods		
Vegetable Lo Mein	½ cup (115 g)	Non-compliant Foods		
Vegetables in creamy or sugary sauces	½ cup (115 g)	Non-compliant Foods		
Yellow squash Chips, commercially made	1 oz (28g)	Non-compliant Foods		
Zucchini Chips, commercially made	1 oz (28g)	Non-compliant Foods		

HEALTH AND NUTRITION WEBSITES

- Centers for Disease Control and Prevention: https://www.cdc.gov/healthyweight
- Fruits and Vegetables Matter: https://www.fruitsandveggiesmatter.gov
- Cooking Light: https://www.cookinglight.com
- Nutrition.gov: https://www.nutrition.gov
- Hormone Foundation: https://www.hormone.org
- American Diabetes Association: https://www.diabetes.org
- American Heart Association: https://www.americanheart.org
- National Institute on Aging: https://www.nia.nih.gov
- National Institutes of Health: http://health.nih.gov
- National Kidney Disease Education Program | NIDDK: https://www.niddk.nih.gov/health-information/community-health-outreach/information-clearinghouses/nkdep
- American Kidney Fund (AKF): https://www.kidneyfund.org/
- The National Institute of Diabetes and Digestive and Kidney Diseases (NIDDK): https://www.niddk.nih.gov/health-information/kidney-disease

ABOUT THE AUTHOR

Dr. H. Maher" is a joint pen name under which Dr. Y. Naitlho, PharmD, and H. Naitlho, MEng (ISAE-SUPAERO), MEng (École de l'Air), MSc (DEA), MBA, co-write books.

Dr. Y. Naitlho, PharmD, has over 25 years of experience in pharmacy practice, with a particular focus on nutrition, healthy eating, and writing. He currently works as a pharmacist and health and nutrition writer, and is an accomplished author of several books in the field of food science, human nutrition, and applied nutrition.

Dr. Y. Naitlho earned his Doctor of Pharmacy degree from the Perm State Pharmaceutical Academy, and he uses his specialized knowledge and experience in nutrition to ensure that the books he co-writes under the pen name "Dr. H. Maher" meet high standards of reliability and integrity. He is committed to creating book designs that cater to readers' dynamic learning needs and to delivering content that is informative and engaging.

H. Naitlho has over 30 years of experience in engineering practice and science and engineering research. He is an accomplished author of several books on business management, as well as a co-author of numerous books on food science, human nutrition, food engineering, and applied nutrition. H. Naitlho holds an Engineering degree from the École Nationale Supérieure d'Aéronautique et de l'Espace (ISAE-SUPAERO), an Engineering degree from the École de l'Air (Salon de Provence), a post-graduate degree in Automatics from Paul Sabatier University, and a further post-graduate degree in Mechanics from Aix

Marseille University, in addition to an MBA from Laureate International Universities.

H. Naitlho's engineering mindset and scientific rigor bring valuable skills to their collaborative work. He is meticulous in refining ideas, analyzing data, and ensuring consistency and attention to detail in their writing projects.

Both Dr. Y. Naitlho and H. Naitlho share a deep passion for helping individuals with diabetes, chronic kidney disease (CKD), and hypertension to live healthier, more fulfilling lives through informed food choices and tailored meal plans. They are dedicated to staying current with the latest research and nutritional guidelines in order to provide their readers with accurate, reliable, and practical information. Their collaborative efforts result in books that empower people with these health conditions to take charge of their health and enjoy a diverse, flavorful diet.

Made in the USA
Las Vegas, NV
21 October 2024

10266429R00223